WHAT READERS ARE SAYING ABOUT
FIT OVER 50

"This book is a lifestyle tour de force. Whether you're trying to figure out which diet to follow, what kind of exercise is best for you, whether to lift weights, how to increase flexibility, how to get the most out of sleep, and dozens of similar questions—you now have an authoritative, comprehensive, holistic, and medically sound handbook for your health. The 22 practical ideas are exactly what I needed to know!"

Patrick Morley, PhD
Executive Chairman, Man in the Mirror, and bestselling author of 21 books,
including *The Man in the Mirror* and *The Christian Man*

"I tend to avoid books that give 'self-help' advice—life is too complicated for easy formulas. The more I went through *Fit over 50*, however, the more I learned. Drawing on the latest research, the authors have assembled a remarkable list of practical suggestions on how to flourish in every way."

Philip Yancey
Author of *Fearfully and Wonderfully: The Marvel of
Bearing God's Image* (with Dr. Paul Brand)

"For those who are interested in a fitness book that deals with the total person: physical, mental, emotional, relational, and spiritual, this is a must read. *Fit over 50* is filled with research-based and biblically sound practical tips for all who want to live life to the fullest."

Gary D. Chapman, PhD, Author of *The 5 Love Languages*

"Wait! Don't let the title fool you. *Fit over 50* is not fiction. This volume is so chockfull of helpful (not to mention up-to-date) advice that I expect it to inform my life for the rest of my days. Walt Larimore and Phillip Bishop manage to keep the cookies on the lower shelf where even we laypeople can reach them. Thoroughly engrossing."

Jerry Jenkins, *New York Times* bestselling author
and owner of the Jerry Jenkins Writers Guild

"God cares about our health—not only for our comfort but for His service. With clear and well-researched advice, Dr. Larimore has fashioned a remarkable guide. With his insightful, whole person understanding of health, he describes practical steps that will fashion our bodies and spirits into the best possible shape to enjoy our health and to serve our King."

Al Weir, MD, President, Christian Medical & Dental Associations

"You may have heard the old saying 'It's not the years in your life that count. It's the life in your years.' In *Fit over 50*, Walt Larimore and Phil Bishop will show you the best way to have *both*."

Jim Daly, President, Focus on the Family

"One of the best all-around books I've ever seen for those of us over 50 who want to improve our all-around health. I'll be putting many of these tips to action in my life and suggesting my friends and colleagues get a copy of their own."

Pat Williams
Senior Vice President of the NBA's Orlando Magic
Author of *Character Carved in Stone*

"What a wonderful resource! It's well-rounded in perspective and grounded in research. *Fit over 50* is an informative read that you will want to keep on your bookshelf for reference long after you've read it. Buy a copy for yourself and one for your friends. They will thank you!"

Juli Slattery, PsyD
President and Cofounder of Authentic Intimacy

"In *Fit over 50* Walt Larimore and Phillip Bishop show you're not here by accident. You were designed; you have a purpose. Their research, knowledge, and practical advice will help you embrace God's gift of life."

Chris Fabry, Author and host of *Chris Fabry Live*

"Walt Larimore is one of those unique physicians who somehow manages to blend both great scientific and technical know-how with incredible empathy and a winsome bedside manner. Who doesn't yearn for that when visiting their doctor? Add to that his theological depth of reflection and concern for the whole person—body and soul—and *Fit over 50* becomes required reading for all of us as we prepare for our final third season of life. It's just good stewardship!"

Scott Bolinder, Executive Director, Institute for Bible Reading

"I am the target audience for this book. I am over 50 and have a strong desire to make simple choices today for a healthier, happier way of life. I have read the book, but I will be keeping it by my side as a go-to reference to keep me on track to be the best me I can be."

Randy Frazee
Lead Pastor, Westside Family Church Lenexa, Kansas and
author of *Real Simplicity: Making Room for Life*

FIT OVER 50

WALT LARIMORE, MD
& PHILLIP BISHOP, EdD

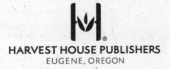

HARVEST HOUSE PUBLISHERS
EUGENE, OREGON

Cover design by Dugan Design Group

Cover photo © Anton Shaparenko; ppvector / Fotolia

Published in association with the literary agency of WordServe Literary Group, Ltd., www.word serveliterary.com.

Fit over 50

Published by Harvest House Publishers
Eugene, Oregon 97408
www.harvesthousepublishers.com

ISBN 978-0-7369-7775 3 (pbk.)
ISBN 978-0-7369-7776-0 (eBook)

Library of Congress Cataloging-in-Publication Data

Names: Bishop, Phillip A., author. | Larimore, Walter L., author.
Title: Fit over 50 : make simple choices today for a healthier, happier you /
    Phillip Bishop and Walt Larimore.
Other titles: Fit over fifty
Description: Eugene, Oregon : Harvest House Publishers, [2019]
Identifiers: LCCN 2018061522 (print) | LCCN 2019001814 (ebook) | ISBN
    9780736977760 (ebook) | ISBN 9780736977753 (paperback)
Subjects: LCSH: Middle-aged persons--Health and hygiene. | Physical fitness
    for older people. | Middle-aged persons--Nutrition. | Middle-aged
    persons--Religious life. | BISAC: RELIGION / Christian Life / Personal
    Growth. | HEALTH & FITNESS / Healthy Living.
Classification: LCC RA777.5 (ebook) | LCC RA777.5 .B57 2019 (print) | DDC
    613.7/0446--dc23
LC record available at https://lccn.loc.gov/2018061522

Printed in the United States of America

19 20 21 22 23 24 25 26 27 / BP-SK / 10 9 8 7 6 5 4 3 2 1

To Bill Judge, my mentor, friend,
and model for health and happiness.

WALT LARIMORE, MD

• • •

To my wife, Brenda, and to Jehovah,
who gives me purpose and meaning!

PROFESSOR EMERITUS PHIL BISHOP, EDD

Disclaimer

This book contains advice and information relating to health and medicine. It is designed for your personal knowledge and to help you be a more informed consumer of medical, dental, and health services. It is not intended to be exhaustive or to replace medical advice from your healthcare professionals and should be used to supplement rather than replace regular care by your physician and others on your healthcare team. Readers are encouraged to consult their healthcare professional with any specific questions and concerns.

All efforts have been made to ensure the accuracy and evidence-based nature of the information contained within this book as of the date published. The endorsers, reviewers, authors, and the publisher expressly disclaim responsibility for any adverse effects resulting from the application of the information contained herein.

The website addresses recommended and cited throughout this book are offered as a resource to you. These websites are not intended in any way to be or imply an endorsement on the part of the authors, the reviewers, the endorsers, or the publisher (Harvest House), nor do we vouch for their content or availability for the life of this book.

CONTENTS

PART ONE:
10 ESSENTIALS

PART TWO:
22 TIPS FOR A HAPPIER, HEALTHIER YOU

Relational Health Tips

Emotional Health Tips

Physical Health Tips

Spiritual Health Tips

MEDICAL ABBREVIATIONS

A1C test	Glycated hemoglobin, glycosylated hemoglobin, hemoglobin A1C, or HbA1C
AAD	American Academy of Dermatology
AAFP	American Academy of Family Physicians
AARP	American Association of Retired Persons
ACG	American College of Gastroenterology
ACS	American Cancer Society
AHA	American Heart Association
ASDS	American Society for Dermatologic Surgery
BCBS	Blue Cross Blue Shield Association
BCC	Basal cell carcinoma
BMI	Body mass index
CBT	Cognitive behavioral therapy
CDC	Centers for Disease Control and Prevention
CL	ConsumerLab or ConsumerLab.com
CRC	Colorectal cancer
DABFM	Diplomat of the American Board of Family Medicine
DASH	Dietary Approaches to Stop Hypertension
DO	Doctor of Osteopathy
DrPH	Doctor of Public Health
EdD	Doctor of Education
ET	Estrogen therapy
FACS	Fellow of the American College of Surgeons
FBS	Fasting blood sugar
FDA	Food and Drug Administration
GSM	Genitourinary syndrome of menopause
HDL	High-density lipoprotein ("good" cholesterol)
Hg	Chemical symbol for mercury
HRS	Health and Retirement Study
HT	Hormone therapy

IFBR	Institute for Bible Reading
JAMA	*Journal of the American Medical Association*
LDL	Low-density lipoprotein ("bad" cholesterol)
MD	Medical Doctor
mg	milligram
NAMS	North American Menopause Society
NHS	National Health Service
NIH	National Institutes of Health
NMCD	Natural Medicines Comprehensive Database
NSAID	Non-steroidal anti-inflammatory drug
NSF	National Sleep Foundation
OSA	Obstructive sleep apnea
PCP	Primary care physician or primary care professional
PCV13	Pneumococcal conjugate vaccine, protects against 13 types of pneumococcal bacteria
PhD	Doctor of Philosophy
PPSV23	Pneumococcal polysaccharides vaccine, protects against 23 types of pneumococcal bacteria
PsyD	Doctor of Psychology
RDN	Registered Dietitian Nutritionist
RET	Resistance exercise training
ROM	Range of motion
R/S	Religion/spirituality
SCC	Squamous-cell carcinoma
SPF	Sun protection factor
Tdap	Tetanus, diphtheria, and acellular pertussis vaccine
US	United States
USP	United States Pharmacopeia
USPSTF	United States Preventive Services Taskforce

FOREWORD

by Dr. David Stevens

You need wisdom, and so do I. In fact, Proverbs 16:16 tells us, "How much better to get wisdom than gold!" (ESV). In *Fit over 50*, the authors have given you a priceless gift that is full of wise insights to prolong your life and increase your happiness.

Wisdom comes from a wealth of knowledge applied well because of an abundance of experience. Walt Larimore and Phil Bishop have both. I love their format for sharing it. They give it to you in small bites, starting with the essentials and then moving to simple-to-understand tips that are practical and easy to apply.

I've been focused on preparing for transitioning out of my position of chief executive officer of the Christian Medical & Dental Associations after 25 years of leading, teaching, and ministering to more than 30,000 healthcare professionals. Recently, I sat down with a financial planner to see if I was prepared not to have a paycheck. If you are over the age of 50, I expect you are thinking about your financial preparation for retirement as well. No matter how well you are prepared, it's not going to do you much good if you're not healthy enough to enjoy it. That's true of your life now as much as it will be then.

When I say healthy, I don't mean just your physical health. This book is going to give you practical tools to also assess how spiritually, relationally, and emotionally healthy you are. The authors offer you proven strategies that will let you be all God intended you to be. If you take what it teaches to heart, it will transform your life.

Ready to start your journey to holistic health?

Find a comfortable chair. Once you start reading, you won't want to stop. Grab a highlighter to mark what you just can't afford to forget. Oh, and make sure you grab a pen as well—not just to make notes but, more importantly, to write your name in the flyleaf. This is the kind of book everyone is going to want to borrow. It's medically accurate, biblically sound, full of great examples, and so very practical. Better yet, because you won't want to take the chance of losing the book that transformed your life, pick up a few extra copies. If you're married, go through it with your spouse. It's one of the most important gifts you could give to a friend. Use it in your small group at church, and you may want to give it to your parents as well.

Countless medically focused self-help books cross my desk. This is one of the absolute best. So here is my prescription for you as you begin. Read one or two chapters a day with a glass of resolve. Chew well and apply each pill of wisdom until your life is revitalized!

• • •

David Stevens, MD, MA (Ethics) is the chief executive officer of the Christian Medical & Dental Associations. He is also the author of *Jesus, M.D.; Leadership Proverbs; Servant Leadership;* and *Beyond Medicine: What Else You Need to Know to Be a Healthcare Missionary.*

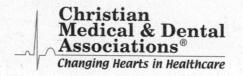

INTRODUCTION

During medical school and a family medicine residency, I* was taught to recognize and treat diseases. I had little training in keeping people healthy and even less in motivating people to become fit and healthy. So, for most of my career, I have had to learn ways to promote health, not just treat sickness. During his training, Phil had much more emphasis on helping folks become healthier, but over the last four decades we have both encountered far too many people who come to us for advice who are highly unhealthy. Many of these people think physical health is the only aspect of health. But if you're in great physical shape and yet suffering emotionally/mentally, relationally, or spiritually, are you highly healthy? You are not!

What motivated you to pick up this book? For what results are you hoping? We hope you desire to be highly healthy in *all* aspects of your life. As evidence-based scientists and educators, we want to teach you how to live better and to live longer—how to become, and stay, fit after age 50. But even more, we want to share lifesaving, life-prolonging, and life-enhancing options for becoming a happier and healthier you by using the latest evidence-based research and the most up-to-date national and international guidelines. Each of our chapters and tips could be expanded into a book of its own. But our prayer is that our introduction to each will fit together like a quilt that you will begin to see the big picture of your design and your Designer.

---

* Even though Walt and Phil wrote this book together, for clarity, *I* will refer to *Walt*, while *we* will refer to *Walt and Phil*.

Of course, we understand that some information in books can become out-of-date quickly with new research being published daily and national guidelines being promulgated and updated frequently. So, to that end, we will be publishing updates to the essentials and tips we're sharing in this book on a frequent basis at www.DrWalt.com/blog. You can either sign up for a free subscription at that site or just return to it every week or two to see what's new.

As followers of Jesus, we know the Bible speaks of us having healthful lives (Deuteronomy 7:12-15; Proverbs 3:7-8; 4:20-22; Jeremiah 33:6). The apostle John wrote, "Dear friend, I pray that you may enjoy good health and that all may go well with you, even as your soul is getting along well" (3 John 1:2). So we'll be infusing our essentials and tips with the eternal truth from God's Word. Because He designed us, we'll be sharing His guidelines for how you can become healthier and happier.

We are not using the terms *happy* or *happier* to mean fortunate, lucky, cheerful, or jovial. The word *happy* in the Bible is much more meaning-ful—it is not an event or occurrence or feeling, but a state that is present even when experiencing a correction from God or enduring hardships (Job 5:17; 1 Peter 3:14; 4:14). *Happy* means *being blessed*. In fact, the word *blessed* used by Jesus in the Sermon on the Mount is derived from the Greek word *makarios*, which also translates to "happy" or "content."

Throughout the book, we'll primarily refer to these three types of large research studies:

- A "review" or "systematic review" answers defined research questions by collecting and summarizing the studies that fit prespecified criteria.

- A "meta-analysis" is the use of statistical methods to summarize the results of multiple clinical studies that fit pre-specified criteria.

- A "randomized controlled trial" (RCT) is a type of scientific experiment that aims to reduce bias when testing an intervention (i.e., a procedure or medication). The people participating in the trial are randomly assigned to either a group receiving a new intervention or to a group receiving either a standard treatment or a placebo. It's often considered the gold standard of human research.

For many footnotes and endnotes on the internet, we have utilized TinyURLs. Just enter the TinyURL into your web browser, and you should be able to find the referenced materials. Any references not available online are cited using standard format.

We have used some primary references, but for medical studies, more often than not we've used trusted secondary resources from medical journalists. These secondary resources not only usually give you a link to the primary resource, they also give you interview quotes from the researchers and other commentators that will help you understand and interpret the data.

Our goal is to use evidence-based, trustworthy, and medically reliable information (no hocus pocus, quick, impossible cures here) while also being biblically sound, so you and your loved ones can live a happy (blessed), healthful life—a lifetime with increased quantity and quality—with eternal life as the ultimate end. Who doesn't want that?

Our prayers for you, as we wrote this book for you, are summed up in these verses that amplify our title and our desires for you:

Fit
Physical training is of some value, but godliness
has value for all things, holding promise for both the
present life and the life to come. (1 Timothy 4:8)

Over 50
Sound the trumpet throughout your land. Consecrate
the fiftieth year...It shall be a jubilee for you...and
is to be holy for you. (Leviticus 25:9-10,12)

Make Simple Choices Today
This day I call the heavens and the earth as witnesses
against you that I have set before you life and death,

blessings and curses. Now choose life, so that you and your children may live. (Deuteronomy 30:19)

For a Healthier

Dear friend, I pray that you may enjoy good health and that all may go well with you, even as your soul is getting along well. (3 John 1:2)

Happier

A happy heart makes the face cheerful...A cheerful heart is good medicine. (Proverbs 15:13; 17:22)

You

As the Father has loved me, so have I loved you. Now remain in my love. If you keep my commands, you will remain in my love...just as I have kept my Father's commands and remain in his love. I have told you this so that my joy may be in you and that your joy may be complete. (John 15:9-11)

So if you're ready, let's get started.

PART ONE

10 ESSENTIALS

1

BALANCE

About ten years ago, I informally surveyed more than 200 physicians and health experts from many countries, asking them:

- What is health?
- What are the essentials of health?
- What tips would you give your friends and family on becoming healthier and living longer?

After cataloging their responses, I searched medical literature, scores of studies, and trustworthy medical recommendations, looking primarily at those focusing on wellness and longevity. Much evidence suggested that living long and well depended on the powerful connection between our physical health and our emotional/mental, relational/family, and spiritual health.[1]

In 2003, I first called these the *four wheels of health*. I proposed that if these four tires were not fully inflated and finely balanced, that one's ride down the road of life would not be as smooth or as long as it could be. And breakdowns could be more frequent than desired. I proposed that of the four wheels of health, the spiritual wheel was the most important because it was connected to the "power steering" Himself.[2] Dr. John Fisher agrees, writing, "At our core, or *coeur*, we humans are spiritual beings…Spiritual health is a, if not THE, fundamental dimension of people's overall health and well-being, permeating and integrating all the other dimensions of health."[3]

Many of the respondents to my survey commented on patients who suffered from poor physical or mental health yet were highly healthy people just because they were so healthy spiritually. One doctor wrote me about a patient who, in the prime of his adult life, became paralyzed from the neck down in an accident, yet who exuded hope and enthusiasm due to his deep relationship with God, supplemented by his rich family and social relationships. The doctor said:

> The essence of true health is physical, emotional, social, and spiritual well-being. When these four dimensions are singing in harmony, you're healthy. That doesn't mean there's no room for a dissonant chord, but that the music of life is pleasant to the ear. My quadriplegic patient seems to me to be highly healthy, despite his sobering physical disability.[4]

I have spoken with many seriously disabled or diseased people who seem healthier than most of my patients. What they all share is a conscious and continuous effort to seek the highest possible degree of health in four aspects of their lives: physical, emotional/mental, relational/social, and spiritual/religious.

Results of a 2018 Harris Poll survey of more than 2,000 American adults examined how people define being healthy. "Ninety-two percent of adults agreed with the statement, 'Health is so much more than just not being sick.' When asked to further define health…[a]mong the factors most frequently cited:[5]

- 59 percent defined it as being happy,
- 56 percent defined it as being calm and relaxed, and
- 53 percent defined it as the ability to live independently."[6]

Interestingly, these four components of health are similar to the definitions given by many experts. One group of experts writes, "Spirituality has now been identified globally as an important aspect for providing answers to many questions related to health and happiness. The World Health Organization is also keen at looking beyond physical, mental and social dimensions of the health, and the member countries are actively exploring the 4th Dimension of the health, i.e. the spiritual health and its impact on the overall health and happiness of an individual."[7]

I defined the four wheels of highly healthy people as:

- *Relational/social health.* The well-being of one's associations with family, friends, and faith in the context of a healthy community.

- *Emotional/mental health.* The well-being of one's mental faculties and one's connection with their emotions.

- *Physical health.* The well-being of one's body.

- *Spiritual health.* The well-being of one's relationship with God.

These four factors continue to be emphasized in the latest scientific research. Harold G. Koenig, MD, a family physician and psychiatrist who is director of the Center for Spirituality, Theology and Health at Duke University, wrote,

> I have reviewed and summarized hundreds of quantitative original data-based research reports examining relationships between religion/spirituality (R/S) and health. These reports have been published in peer-reviewed journals in medicine, nursing, social work, rehabilitation, social sciences, counseling, psychology, psychiatry, public health, demography, economics, and religion. The majority of studies report significant relationships between R/S and better health.[8]

The Oxford University *Handbook of Religion and Health* exhaustively documents thousands of peer-reviewed studies reporting the direct relationships between R/S and physical, emotional, and social health.[9] Family physician Wayne Jonas, MD, says, "As physicians we should be asking, 'What matters?' instead of just, 'What's the matter?'"[10]

English cleric and theologian John Wesley (1703–1791), a cofounder of Methodism, wanted his family, friends, and followers to enjoy healthy lives. In 1747 he penned "Primitive Physick, or An Easy and Natural Method of Curing Most Diseases."[11] He defines *physic* as "the art of healing."[12] In this treatise he suggested 37 rules for living a balanced life and preventing disease—rules that involve all four wheels of health. These are my favorites:

1. People should have those who…are much about them (who are) sound, sweet, and healthy.

2. Water is the wholesomest of all drinks.

3. Persons should eat very light suppers and that two or three hours before going to bed.

4. Constantly go to bed about nine and rise at four or five.

5. A due degree of exercise is indispensably necessary to health and long life. Walking is the best exercise…The open air, when the weather is fair, contributes much to the benefit of exercise.

6. Those who read or write much, should learn to do it standing; otherwise, it will impair their health.

7. Exercise first, should be always on an empty stomach; secondly, should never be continued to weariness; thirdly, after it, we should take to cool by degrees.

8. The slow and lasting passions, such as grief and hopeless love, bring on chronical diseases.

9. Till the passion which caused the disease is calmed, medicine is applied in vain.

10. The love of God, as it is the sovereign remedy of all miseries…and by the unspeakable joy and perfect calm serenity and tranquility it gives the mind; it becomes the most powerful of all the means of health and long life.

These four wheels are also outlined in the Bible, where Luke, the only physician who authored a book in the Bible (and he wrote two books, the Gospel of Luke and Acts), observed, "Jesus grew in wisdom (emotional/mental health) and stature (physical health), and in favor with

God (spiritual health) and man (relational/social health)" (Luke 2:52). Of course, we added the parentheticals, but they make sense, don't they?

How many people have we met (other than Jesus) who have all four wheels perfectly balanced? None. Not a single person! The important thing to remember is that we all share a common need to constantly balance the different parts of our life. Maintaining a highly healthy balance is a lifelong and life-enhancing task.

Unfortunately, simply scrutinizing these pages won't produce results. To become a highly healthy person, you'll need to understand the four wheels of health and then take personal responsibility for your health. You'll be tempted to neglect what is needed to become highly healthy. It takes work. It takes time. You may be enticed by some healthcare scammers who promise that their particular therapy, tonic, or tablet will simply, easily, and quickly cure all that ails you. It won't.

But we have tried to make this work easier, more enjoyable, and more effective by identifying for you ten essentials and dozens of tips for highly healthy living after age 50 that encompass all four wheels of health. Of course, there are many, many more tips we have not included, but we believe the ones we have chosen are some of the most important and helpful. As a result, our prayer is that you will consider and apply as many as you can.

Now, to start, we will share a tool to help you assess and measure the current status of each of your four health wheels. Visit DrWalt.com and scroll to the bottom of the page where you'll see a link to Assessment Tools and Websites. Print off the 4 Wheel Diagram—Adult,[13] and click on either:

1. "Assess Your Health—Adult."[14]

2. "Assess Your Health—Christian."[15] The latter has a more robust spiritual history for Christians.

It can take up to an hour to take and grade the assessments, but when you're finished, you'll have an accurate picture of your four health wheels. Are any flat? Out of balance? In need of a tune-up? If so, this book is for you!

2

PREVENTIVE CARE

For millennia, the only tool physicians utilized for health promotion was called *secondary prevention*, where a physician saw a patient, treated a disease, and then attempted, secondarily, to prevent worsening or recurrence. But now it is widely accepted that *primary prevention* is the most effective and arguably economical strategy in healthcare. Many choices and behaviors are associated with dramatic increases in length of life and quality of life—especially by preventing or delaying chronic debilitating diseases such as obesity, diabetes, heart disease, stroke, and cancer. In other words, you can often prevent disease before it starts with *primary prevention*. It boils down to a series of choices you, your family, and loved ones will make on a day-to-day basis.[1]

I once had a patient tell me, "Doc, I've just got poor genes. Everyone in my family has died young. Guess I will also." I explained to him that a long, high-quality life is not solely a result of good genetics. Sure, genes are important, but even more important are the decisions we make about daily lifestyle issues—sleeping, diet, exercise, work, leisure, meditation, prayer, reducing stress, and improving relationships. About 20 years ago, some experts believed that as much as 70 to 80 percent of what controls our lifespan was related to our lifestyle, not our genes. In other words, genetics only accounted for 20 to 30 percent of an individual's chance of surviving to old age.[2] A 2018 study in the journal *Genetics* reported that "genes accounted for well under 7 percent of people's life span, versus the 20 to 30 percent of most previous estimates."[3]

The five leading causes of death in the United States are heart disease, cancer, chronic lower respiratory diseases (such as emphysema and chronic bronchitis), stroke, and accidental injuries. For persons aged 80 years or less, these represented nearly 900,000 deaths in 2010 according to the Centers for Disease Control and Prevention (CDC). The good news is that nearly a quarter (more than 200,000) of these deaths are considered preventable—in other words, they are premature deaths that could have been avoided.[4]

Another study by the Harvard School of Public Health examined the reversible risk factors for premature death in the US. Here are the estimated numbers of premature lives lost annually—virtually all of which could have been be prevented, reversed, or treated:[5]

1. smoking: 467,000

2. high blood pressure: 395,000

3. overweight/obesity: 216,000

4. inadequate physical activity/inactivity: 191,000

5. high blood sugar: 190,000

6. high LDL (low-density lipoprotein) or "bad" cholesterol: 113,000

In late 2018, a first-of-its-kind measurement by the Blue Cross Blue Shield Association (BCBS) pinpointed, by county, what is impacting Americans' health both by lowering quality and quantity of life. The top five health conditions that have the greatest impact include:[6]

1. *Hypertension—National Health Impact 12.5 percent.* More commonly known as *high blood pressure*, it can cause heart attack or stroke and is also known as *the silent killer* because it has no early noticeable symptoms but creates an extra load on the heart and blood vessels.

2. *Major Depression— National Health Impact 9 percent.* Depression frequently goes undiagnosed or untreated.

3. *High Cholesterol—National Health Impact 8.6 percent.*

High cholesterol can be hereditary or from the result of unhealthy diet and lifestyle choices and can increase the risk of heart attack and stroke.

4. *Coronary Artery Disease — National Health Impact 7 percent.* High blood pressure, high cholesterol, smoking, and diabetes can all damage or obstruct the inner layer of coronary arteries, which, over time, can worsen and become coronary artery disease, putting you at much higher risk of heart attack.

5. *Type 2 Diabetes—National Health Impact 5.5 percent.* In people with diabetes, blood sugar levels rise higher than normal. Type 2 diabetes, the most common form of the disease, is caused by obesity and lack of physical activity in about 90 percent of cases.

Once again, the many lifestyle tips we're going to teach you can prevent many and help treat almost all of these disorders. To learn more about the health issues impacting your county or state, take a tour on the interactive BCBS Health Index map at tinyurl.com/y6oyrfpv.

The National Research Council and Institute of Medicine report that up to half of all premature deaths in the US are attributable to behavioral and other preventable factors—including modifiable habits such as tobacco use, poor diet, and lack of exercise.[7] A 2018 study from the CDC found "heart disease is the leading cause of death among American adults" and "heart problems that were largely preventable (including heart attacks, strokes, heart failure) killed around 415,000 Americans" in 2016.[8]

The number one killer of women is heart disease, accounting for about one in every four female deaths. Despite increases in public awareness over the past decade,[9] only one in five American women believe heart disease is their greatest health threat.[10] Many women believe breast cancer is their major health concern when, in fact, this disease is far down the list. In reality, more women die of cardiovascular disease than all cancers put together.[11] For example, only about 1 in 31 deaths of women is caused by breast cancer.[12]

Breast cancer is an appropriate concern for women, and we've devoted an entire tip to it. But our point is that cardiovascular disease should be of even *more* concern because 90 percent of women have one or more risk factors for developing heart disease or stroke.[13] Almost two-thirds of women who die suddenly of coronary heart disease have no symptoms.[14]

As simple a choice as improving your nutrition can have substantial benefits. According to one report, "A diet quality score based on the PURE study, which advocates eating more of seven key foods—fruits, vegetables, nuts, legumes, fish, dairy, and non-processed red meat—has been linked to lower premature deaths and reduced cardiovascular events such as heart attack and stroke in at least three large independent studies."[15]

Smoking is a major factor in four of the five leading causes of death: heart disease, cancer, lung disease, and stroke. Smoking one to five cigarettes a day increases heart attack risk by 38 percent—40 cigarettes a day increases risk by 900 percent.[16] In a 2017 study of more than 235,000 adults aged 59 to 82, the National Institutes of Health (NIH) found smokers who smoked one to ten cigarettes per day had more than twice the risk of developing a tobacco-related cancer (such as lung, bladder, or pancreatic cancer). Even less than one cigarette a day almost doubled the risks of these cancers. The NIH concluded, "Even low-levels of cigarette smoking causes cancer" and *all* smokers "would benefit from cessation."[17]

Data from 52 countries reported that nine factors (abnormal lipids, smoking, hypertension, diabetes, abdominal obesity, psychosocial factors, low consumption of fruits and vegetables, alcohol use, and low regular physical activity) account for most of the risk of cardiovascular disease worldwide.[18] This huge study also found that stress—whether at home or at work, finances, or major life events—although less dangerous to our health than smoking, was as bad as high blood pressure or abdominal obesity.[19] The minimal lifestyle intervention that has been suggested to be healthful for stress reduction is 10 to 20 minutes a day of silence, relaxation, prayer, or meditation.[20]

"This makes sense, and I want to improve my health," you may say, "but why buy another book on health? Can't I just find all this on the internet?" Not necessarily. In fact, one group of researchers found that among health websites, retail websites presenting information on products they were selling had the lowest level of medical accuracy (only 9 percent). On the other hand, government websites (.gov) and websites of national organizations (.org) had the highest level of accuracy (81 and 73 percent, respectively). Note that even these "reputable" sources weren't close to 100 percent accurate![21]

Shockingly, educational websites (.edu sites, e-books, peer-reviewed articles) only had 50 percent accurate medical information. The majority of the books found by search engines either provided outdated or irrelevant information. Blogs and websites of individuals are even worse, having low rates of accuracy (26 and 30 percent, respectively).[22]

The American Academy of Family Physicians (AAFP) reported in 2018 that 97 percent of family physicians polled said they have had patients come to an office visit with inaccurate medical information from an online source.[23] Another study by researchers from Harvard Medical School and Boston's Children's Hospital found internet symptom checkers varied widely in accuracy. On average, they included the correct diagnosis in the first three results only 51 percent of the time. Individual symptom checkers ranged from 34 percent to 84 percent accurate. Overall, the chances of finding the right diagnosis listed first were poor. On the low end, one checker listed the correct condition first only 5 percent of the time, whereas the best only listed it 50 percent of the time. Understandably, the sites did better at identifying common conditions than uncommon ones.[24] Therefore, when researching health conditions or treatments online or in books (including this one) or magazines, your best bet is to always check the advice with your physician or pharmacist.

Our prayer is that you come to understand and appreciate the great privilege of stewardship you have in becoming and remaining a highly healthy person. Family history and genetics play a role, to be sure, but it is increasingly obvious that your lifestyle decisions play a much larger role.

The Bible teaches that it is our sacred duty to be proactive about our own self-care. God considers the human body, which He designed, to be His temple. "Do you not know that your bodies are temples of the Holy Spirit, who is in you, whom you have received from God? You are not your own; you were bought at a price. Therefore, honor God with your bodies" (1 Corinthians 6:19-20). This book was written to help you do just this by giving you medically trustworthy and biblically sound advice that is reliable, reputable, and reproducible to help you and your family live longer and higher quality lives.

Many of our tips grow out of what I have called the *Ten Commandments of Preventive Medicine*.[25] We could identify several more tips related to preventing disease, but these should get us off to an excellent start. And, of course, we'll be adding other tips for your physical, emotional/mental, relational/social, and spiritual health.

1. See a primary care physician for regular preventive maintenance and care.

2. Avoid or reduce obesity.

3. Exercise regularly—and wisely.

4. Pursue a lifelong monogamous marriage relationship.

5. Protect your dental health.

6. Be careful with alcohol.

7. Stay away from tobacco.

8. Reduce unnecessary stress.

9. Double-check alternative health approaches with your physician or pharmacist.

10. Use automobile safety devices and install and maintain smoke detectors and carbon monoxide detectors in your home.

You may not find a lot of surprises in these first ten tips—but the real questions are these:

• To which of these guidelines do you need to begin paying attention?

- When do you plan to start implementing some of these tips?
- What strategies will ensure your success?

A colleague of mine has suggested a simple formula for good health: 0-5-10-30-150. Zero cigarettes; five servings of fruit and vegetables a day; 10 minutes of silence, relaxation, meditation, or prayer a day; a body mass index (BMI) of less than 30; and 150 minutes of exercise per week. We'll have more tips for you in each of these areas.[26]

Primary prevention is not the only critical aspect of maintaining and improving your health; screening for early disease and vaccinations against disease is also lifesaving. A 2018 study revealed some shocking information.[27] Only 8 percent of US adults age 35 and older had received all high-priority recommended preventive services. Five percent of adults did not receive any such services. How many of the following 13 services have you had? Men (♂) should have up to 11, while women (♀) should have up to 13.

PERCENTAGE OF US ADULTS (> 35 YEARS OLD) RECEIVING RECOMMENDED PREVENTIVE SERVICES[28]

SCREENING	
Blood Pressure	87%
Breast Cancer (♀)	74%
Cervical Cancer (♀)	68-75%
Cholesterol	82%
Colon Cancer (> 45 y/o)	64%
Osteoporosis (♀)	63%
SCREENING AND COUNSELING	
Alcohol Use	41%

Depression	41%
Obesity	64%
Tobacco Use	62%
VACCINATIONS	
Influenza (Flu)	49%
Zoster (Shingles)	38%
Pneumococcal (Pneumonia)	66%

Don't be surprised if you had a low score. A 2018 study by the National Cancer Institute (NCI) found Americans lack understanding of cancer screening. In fact, only about one in twenty folks answered correctly four true-false questions about cancer screening.[29] This suggested that "most people have inaccurate beliefs about what cancer screening tests can do and what they cannot." The NCI's lead author remarked, "That's a little bit alarming," adding, "We just haven't done a good job in educating the public about these nuances in cancer screening that are important to understand."[30] But, our tips will help you grasp these lifesaving concepts.

We hope that this book will help you increase your knowledge and assist you in making wise decisions about your health. By beginning with a single step and continuing to improve on a day-to-day basis, you, your family, and your loved ones will be on your way to not only becoming happier and healthier but living longer.

3

FORGIVENESS

All of us have been wronged—have experienced unjust wounds. Unfortunately, some of us allow these hurts to grow into chronic anger, hostility, bitterness, grudges, cynicism, contempt, resentment, hatred, or victimhood we can't, or won't, leave behind. We are either unwilling or unable to get beyond our pain. We don't understand that our unforgiveness is a slow, lethal toxin, poisoning us from the inside out. It's not a small problem. Sixty-two percent of American adults say they need more forgiveness in their personal lives, according to a survey by the Fetzer Institute.[1]

For anyone who has suffered as a result of another's actions, we have this prescription: *Make peace with your past.* You must undertake the daunting task of learning to accept what you cannot change and let go of your pain and anger arising from the ways you have been hurt. In fact, your life may depend on it.

One group of researchers reported that those who held grudges had higher rates of heart disease and cardiac arrest, elevated blood pressure, stomach ulcers, arthritis, back problems, headaches, and chronic pain than those who didn't.[2] Johns Hopkins experts tell us that people who hold grudges are more likely to experience severe depression and post-traumatic stress disorder.[3] A Berkley study found that when people recalled a grudge, their blood pressure spiked.[4]

"There is an enormous physical burden to being hurt and disappointed," says Karen Swartz, MD, from Johns Hopkins Hospital. "Chronic anger puts you into a fight-or-flight mode, which results in numerous changes in heart rate, blood pressure and immune response. Those changes, then, increase the risk of depression, heart disease and diabetes, among other conditions. Forgiveness, however, calms stress levels, leading to improved health."[5]

The good news is research that shows the simple act of forgiveness "can reap huge rewards for your health, lowering the risk of heart attack; improving cholesterol levels and sleep; and reducing pain, blood pressure, and levels of anxiety, depression and stress. And research points to an increase in the forgiveness-health connection as you age."[6]

Harboring anger, hurt, or resentment always gnaws away at a person's happiness and health. A 2014 review article concluded, "In an era of lawsuits, it can sometimes seem like forgiveness is a concept from biblical times. But a wealth of research suggests we should apply the act to our daily lives because it may hold a myriad of health benefits."[7] Another researcher concluded, "Failing to forgive, or unforgiveness, is the practice of engaging in ruminative thoughts of anger, vengeance, hate, and resentment that have unproductive outcomes for the ruminator, such as increased anxiety, depression, elevated blood pressure, vascular resistance, decreased immune response, and worse outcomes in coronary artery disease."[8]

On the other hand, according to Mayo Clinic, forgiveness "brings with it plenty of health benefits, including improved relationships, decreased anxiety and stress, lower blood pressure, a lowered risk of depression, and stronger immune and heart health. Letting go of negative emotions can often have a remarkable impact on the body."[9] The American Psychological Association says, "Forgiveness can improve mental and physical health."[10] Dr. J. Nick Pitts writes, "When we fail to free others from the pain they caused us, we continue to hold ourselves captive to the pain that hurts us."[11] It's as if the experts are all saying, "Forgive to live!"

If you're one of the many folks who believe the old adage, "To err is human, to forgive divine," take note that medical science is establishing that "To err is human, but to forgive is highly healthy." Unforgiveness (and its toxic ABCs: anger, bitterness, and cynicism) are among the negative moods that can be lethal. According to ScienceAlert,

"Researchers found that people's negative moods…were associated with higher levels of inflammation—the body's natural immune response to injury and infection, but which is also a common hallmark of ill health and chronic disease."[12]

If you want to be highly healthy, you have to admit that although you may have been wronged, you've also been wrong to foster your anger, bitterness, shame, or regrets, and to withhold your forgiveness. Admitting you were wrong to hold on to these emotions is a form of confession.

In the Bible, to *confess* is simply to agree with God that certain attitudes, emotions, or actions are wrong. We can begin to find healing when we simply agree we missed the mark, that we fell short. The Bible teaches, "If we confess our sins, [God] is faithful and just and will forgive us our sins and purify us from all unrighteousness" (1 John 1:9).

Ninety-four percent of Americans believe forgiveness is good, but only 48 percent admit they usually tried to forgive.[13] Dr. Pitts observes, "As many have said before, holding a grudge is like drinking poison and hoping the other person dies. A grudge offers us the chance at vindication, but it overpromises and under delivers. In the biblical narrative, we read how bitterness takes root (Hebrews 12:15). Instead of letting it take root, don't let the sun go down on the wrong (Ephesians 4:26)."[14]

Knowing that the Creator of the universe, who designed each of us, is willing and able to completely forgive all of our past wrongs allows us to begin the process of forgiving. Jesus made this clear when He taught, "If you hold anything against anyone, forgive them, so that your Father in heaven may forgive you your sins" (Mark 11:25). He modeled this by asking God the Father to forgive those who were sneering at Him and mocking Him—even His executioners (Luke 23:34).

Theologian and missionary Danny Loe writes, "It has been a very powerful help in my life that when I am faced with needing to forgive someone I would just as soon *not* forgive, that God has reminded me of Ephesians 4:32 [Be kind and compassionate to one another, forgiving each other, just as in Christ God forgave you]. I forgive because I have been forgiven." He adds, "Paul makes it clear here that the *ability* to forgive is based on the *fact* that we have been forgiven."[15]

If you need to confess any wrong to God, do so—knowing that with this confession comes forgiveness and cleansing. Afterward, thank God that He has forgiven your wrongdoing. You exhale (confess) the bad, and then inhale the good (the forgiveness of God).[16] It's a form of spiritual breathing.

Then, if someone has wronged you and you've never forgiven them, make the conscious decision to forgive them. You may even want to consider visiting or calling them to confess the anger or bitterness that has been in your heart and tell them you've forgiven them. They may not choose to receive the forgiveness, but if you're giving it sincerely and with a pure heart, it will improve your health and set you free.

In His Sermon on the Mount, Jesus taught, "If you are offering your gift at the altar and there remember that your brother has something against you, leave your gift there in front of the altar. First go and be reconciled to your brother; then come and offer your gift" (Matthew 5:23-24). Even if the fault is with the other person, it is *your* responsibility to attempt to heal the relationship.

We hope you are beginning to see that unforgiveness is lethal. On the one hand, you may be harboring resentment for a wrong done to you, but on the other hand, you may fail at asking forgiveness from others whom you have wronged. In that case, it's your responsibility to go to them (or contact them if you can't go in person) to admit your wrong and ask for forgiveness. One of my pastors teaches, "I encourage people to ask simple yes or no questions when seeking forgiveness. The simple question, 'Will you forgive me?' requires a definitive yes or no and leaves no wiggle room for later doubt, especially when the reply is, 'Yes, I forgive you.'"

Of course, sometimes reconciliation is impossible, even with the wise guidance of a Christian pastor or counselor. And sometimes resolution or restitution is impossible due to ongoing abuse or violence. In cases like these, you can pray for the people from whom you're estranged and then leave the rest to God. Fix whatever is wrong if you can.

However, *if* you are at fault, apologize. Accept any consequences that may result. Make restitution.

The bottom line is, that to the extent it is possible on your part, banish grudges and resentments—to let them go so you can be set free. Make the *conscious choice* to forgive—even knowing that you may have to practice forgiveness over and over.

Promise to forgive those who hurt you. Understand, though, that it may be difficult to forgive and forget. Rarely can one *completely* forget what happened. Don't even try. But prayerfully, over time, you'll perhaps less often recall and brood over the injustice and hurt. It has been wisely said, "The first to apologize is the bravest, the first to forgive is the strongest, the first to forget is the happiest."

According to the researchers at the Greater Good Science Center at the University of California, Berkeley, "Forgiveness is the act of consciously deciding to let go of resentment or vengeance toward another entity who has harmed you in some way (whether or not they're deserving of that forgiveness)." They add, "It does not mean having to forget or condone the wrongdoing committed against you."[17] Forgiving is a decision—an act of your will—but restoration of trust, by contrast, is conditional and takes time. The two are not the same.

It's worth repeating one more time: Forgiving someone for something they have done against you, or to you, does *not* condone or sanction their behavior. It does not excuse them from their actions or even the consequences of their wrongs. It doesn't mean you shouldn't be cautious when interacting with this person. This complex process of forgiving can be less daunting with the help of a licensed counselor or therapist. Focus on the Family can assist you in finding counselors in your area. (You can reach Focus on the Family at 1-800-A-FAMILY or at tinyurl.com/ya3f8eo9.)

Making forgiveness a habit takes practice. In our experience, the emotional and spiritual healing that comes from forgiveness can only begin after someone makes the decision to forgive and follows through with that decision. Once the healing process begins, you'll begin to notice changes. Researchers tell us the changes forgivers experience filter into their beliefs, behaviors, and body and brain biochemistry. Even their facial expressions, posture, and body language can change. Their blood pressure and heart function are likely to improve. Bottom line—forgiveness can heal both the person who is forgiven and the person who forgives.

Forgivers often come to realize how their pain and suffering has resulted in positive transformation as they begin to witness seedlings of *good* growing out of the ashes of hurt and the ruins of burned-out dreams. Many even begin to feel a twinge of joy for the suffering they've experienced—they are able to cultivate gratitude for past pain. For the person who has a personal relationship with God and who is growing spiritually, it is indeed possible—in fact, probable—that gratitude, even for suffering, will develop. The apostle Paul taught this principle: "Just as you received Christ Jesus as Lord, continue to live in him, rooted and built up in him, strengthened in the faith as you were taught, and overflowing with thankfulness" (Colossians 2:6-7). Highly healthy people become thankful people—full of a gratitude that overflows—even in the midst of pain and suffering.

Research indicates that individuals who perform acts of kindness such as forgiveness receive a boost in life satisfaction.[18] Another study found that even remembering a past act of kindness boosted levels of happiness in the present.[19] Various studies conclude that random acts of kindness can improve your well-being,[20] increase energy levels,[21] and lower stress.[22] In other words, kindness to others is actually kindness to yourself.

The final phase of forgiving involves using your healing to reach out to others—to comfort them in their pain. The apostle Paul found this to be true in his life. He wrote, "God…comes alongside us when we go through hard times, and before you know it, he brings us alongside someone else who is going through hard times so that we can be there for that person just as God was there for us" (2 Corinthians 1:3-4 MSG).

To become a highly healthy person, you must practice acceptance and letting go. You must practice forgiving. It has been said that justice is giving to others what they deserve; mercy is not giving what is deserved; grace is giving what is not deserved. Highly healthy people are liberal dispensers of mercy and grace. By becoming a forgiver, your heart, spirit, and soul will be healthier.

4

REDUCE S-A-D-NESS

Stress, anxiety, and depression (under the umbrella of what I have called *S-A-D-ness*[1]) are ubiquitous. In fact, reports tell us that "more Americans than ever before are suffering from stress, anxiety, and depression."[2] The most recent annual measure by Gallup of its *Negative Experience Index*, which annually tracks people's experiences, reported that stress, anxiety, and depression—overall unhappiness—is at an unprecedented and all-time high.[3]

Truth be told, we all can have one or more of these negative experiences to some degree most every day. But, when one or more of them grow too heavy, they can begin to have surprisingly negative effects—not only on our emotional health but also on our physical, relational, and spiritual health. To lighten your load for the difficult journey of life, we'll examine each one and show you how to evaluate your level.

Evaluating Stress

Stress is unavoidable in contemporary life. In one Gallup survey, about eight in ten Americans say they frequently (44 percent) or sometimes (35 percent) encounter stress in their daily lives.[4] I can't tell you how many of my patients have told me that they feel as if they are running about as fast as they can on the hamster wheel of life. Nearly all of them report they feel "super stressed."

Stress can come from big things—retirement, job change, pregnancy, a new grandbaby, moving, the loss of a loved one, attending a new school, or beginning a new job. Stress can also come from little things—a surprise schedule change, a change in the weather, a flat tire or traffic jam, a sudden deadline, misplaced keys, or an electrical outage. These events are *stressors*. We'll use the words *stress* and *stressors* to mean the same thing.

Some stress is good. *Eustress* is the term for normal stress that is beneficial or good stress. *Distress* refers to harmful stress.[5] We are designed to act in response to certain amounts of stress. It can help us grow—physically, emotionally, relationally, and spiritually. In the physical realm, our body is in constant flux. For example, our bones are constantly being dissolved and new bone being laid down. With the right amount of stress, our bones become thicker and stronger. We improve our strength and cardiovascular fitness by means of properly apportioned eustress. In the mental and emotional realm, certain amounts of stress keep our mind and emotions healthy. Spiritually, we are constantly being tested—stressed—by our Creator. This "refining" is one path to improved spiritual health. Our point is simple: Stress is not only normal—it's necessary.

However, too much distress at one single time or for too long a time (*chronic stress*) can lead to significant weakness in our overall well-being. Most of us are created with the capacity to handle a certain amount of stress—our *stress bucket*, so to speak. Some have small buckets and others have larger buckets. No matter what our capacity for coping with stress, if there's too much stress and our bucket overflows, stress spills over and can damage our health.[6]

Mayo Clinic experts say, "Stress that's left unchecked can contribute to many health problems, such as high blood pressure, heart disease, obesity and diabetes. Common effects of stress on your body include headache, muscle tension or pain, chest pain, fatigue, change in sex drive, stomach upset, sleep problems."[7] Too much stress will not only keep you from becoming a highly healthy person, but it may also prematurely kill you.

A recent study published in *Heart Rhythm* reported "that increased stress levels associated with today's hectic lifestyles were linked to an increased likelihood of sudden cardiac arrest any time of day, any day of the week."[8] The study's lead investigator, Dr. Sumeet Chugh, a professor of medicine and medical director of the Heart Rhythm Center at the Smidt Heart Institute at Cedars-Sinai, said, "We now live in a fast-paced, 'always on' era that causes increased psychosocial stress and…an increase in the likelihood of sudden cardiac arrest."[9]

So what about you? Are there too many stressors in your life? You won't know until you check your stress level. Just as you may not know your car's oil level is getting low unless you check the dip stick, the same is true for stress, anxiety, and depression. But, by finding this out early, before the problem worsens, it's easier to prevent a major breakdown. Several free, easy-to-use stress evaluation tools are available:

- NYSUT Stress Assessments (uses "Symptoms of Stress," "Perceived Stress Scale," and "The Ardell Wellness Stress Test" measurements)— tinyurl.com/yanh78r7
- Holmes and Rahe Stress Scale—tinyurl.com/odoejud
- Mental Health America Stress Test—tinyurl.com/y6wubdrc

If you scored high on one of these screening tools, reducing your daily stress will contribute to becoming more highly healthy. Here are a few ways to reduce stress:

- Taking short walks with a friend or a loved one, your spouse or kids, for just 30 minutes per day—and it does not have to be all at one time—can help improve your sleep, boost your mood, and reduce stress. My friend Rob Person calls it "taking time to kick the leaves."

- Try taking emotional health breaks every two or three hours. Think of something you like to do—read, journal, walk, meditate, sing, listen to music, pray, take a yoga or stretch break, read and memorize Scripture—and do it, even if only for a few minutes. When I was a young husband, I often brought my stress home. My mentor, dairyman Bill Judge, taught me to stop at a park on the way home and take a short walk to "dump my stress in a nearby stream." This simple technique allowed me to chunk my distress and not carry it home, where it could be noxious.

- Set goals and priorities. Studies consistently show that people with clear goals outperform people with vague aspirations.[10] Decide what God is calling you to do—what must get done and what can wait. My friend Reverend Rodney Wood says, "You have exactly the right amount of time to do all that God has called you to do. However, you do not have enough time to do God's calling as well as those things that are not God's calling for you."[11]

- Learn to say no to new tasks if they are putting you into overload or if God is not clearly calling you to them. Christian Counselor Barb Seeds says, "In managing one's stress level, I would suggest to a client that before adding something to their plate, that they take a few minutes to write down how the additional activity would impact their schedule, their family's other activities, the overall rhythm of the home. And, if they already have children's sports activities, Bible studies, etc., how those responsibilities would be affected."[12]

- Note what you have accomplished at the end of the day, not what you have been unable to do. Stay connected with people who can provide emotional and other support. To reduce stress, ask for help from friends, family, and your faith community.

- British research showed reading was the most effective way to overcome stress. It took the average person just six minutes to relax once they started turning pages, and it reduced stress levels 68 percent.[13]

If none of these options helps, consider exploring stress coping programs in your community. Seek the advice and assistance of a trusted pastoral professional or a Christian mental health expert. God never promised us a comfortable life (2 Timothy 3:12; 1 Peter 4:12) but to comfort us in this life (John 16:33; 2 Corinthians 1:2-4).

Evaluating Anxiety

We all know what it's like to feel anxious. Do you remember the butterflies in your stomach before a first date or a big presentation, the tension you feel when someone is angry with you, the way your heart pounds when you're in danger? Anxiety in its most basic form is healthy—a normal response designed by our Creator to arouse us and get us ready for action. Anxiety can prepare you physically and emotionally for a threatening situation. Anxiety caused us to study harder for our exams; it's what keeps us on our toes when we're giving a speech or teaching. Anxiety is designed both to help us cope and to assist us in performing at a higher level.

An anxiety disorder is another matter. The disorder occurs when anxiety does the opposite of what it was designed to do. Instead of helping you cope, it prevents you from coping and dramatically disrupts your daily life. Anxiety disorders aren't just a case of bad nerves. They are illnesses that often have roots in both our biological and biochemical makeup and our past experiences. Not surprisingly, anxiety disorders frequently run in families. For some who live with this disorder, the anxious feelings may be so uncomfortable that to avoid them they stop some, or most, of their everyday accomplishments. Others self-medicate with alcohol, drugs, or frantic activities. For others, panic attacks can occur so swiftly and strongly they result in experiences of terror, which can completely immobilize them.

Of all the emotional health maladies, anxiety disorders are the most common and pervasive in the US.[14] Nearly 40 million Americans experience an anxiety disorder in any given year.[15] There are several types of anxiety disorders, each with its own distinct features and its own treatment. Many people, especially those of religious conviction, believe people should be able to overcome the symptoms by sheer willpower or by more faithful observance of religious ritual or practice. However, for people with these disorders, this simply is not the case. The good news is that effective new treatments are available.

If you frequently experience anxiety—and even if you aren't sure whether you do or don't—there are several free, easy-to-use anxiety evaluation tools that allow you to check your "oil level" when it comes to anxiety:

- Zung Self-Rated Anxiety Scale—tinyurl.com/y9srp2sx
- Hamilton Anxiety Rating Scale—tinyurl.com/ycpvf7mj

You can find a number of other Anxiety Tests here—tinyurl.com/ydchqfoo.

The purpose of this section is not to discuss these specific disorders or their treatments in depth, but rather to convince you that if your emotional wheel is not strong, you can strengthen it. If you don't work to improve it, it's less likely you'll become a highly healthy person. But we do want to briefly discuss the most common of the anxiety disorders—one called *generalized anxiety disorder* (GAD). People with GAD worry at length about health, money, job, family, or work. Simply the thought of getting through the day provokes anxiety. They are unable to relax and often have trouble falling or staying asleep. Their worries are typically accompanied by physical symptoms—especially trembling, twitching, muscle tension, headaches, irritability, sweating, or hot flashes. They may feel light-headed or out of breath. They may feel nauseated or have to go to the bathroom frequently. They may have palpitations or chest pain. Sometimes they feel as though they have a lump in their throat. They tend to feel tired, have trouble concentrating, and sometimes suffer depression.[16] If anxiety is negatively affecting you or those around you, consider seeing your family physician, a licensed pastoral professional, or a Christian counselor. Experts recommend, "Anxiety disorders should be treated with psychological therapy, pharmacotherapy, or a combination of both. Cognitive behavioral therapy can be regarded as the psychotherapy with the highest level of evidence."[17]

Evaluating Depression

Depression is the second most common issue that can weaken emotional health and prevent people from staying highly healthy. It often accompanies anxiety disorders, and when it does, it should be treated along with the anxiety.[18] Depression may be accompanied by feelings of sadness, apathy, and hopelessness, as well as by changes in appetite or sleep. Depression can also make it difficult to concentrate.

According to National Alliance on Mental Illness contributor Dr. Beth Salcedo, "When a person experiences two or more illnesses at the same time, those illnesses are called *comorbid*… In mental health, one of the more common comorbidities is that of depression and anxiety. Some estimates show that 60 percent of those with anxiety will also have symptoms of depression, and the numbers are similar for those with depression also experiencing anxiety."[19]

Researchers tell us much of what manifests as depression is caused by an imbalance in the hormones of the brain. A 2018 study revealed 37 percent of adults take medications that actually increase the risk of depression, "including hormones, blood pressure medications, and medicines for heartburn."[20] Regardless of the cause, most depression is treatable with a variety of treatments—anti-depression medications, dietary supplements, nutritional therapies, exercise, light therapy, pastoral counseling, or psychotherapy. "Up to 80% of those treated for depression show an improvement in their symptoms within four to six weeks of beginning medication, psychotherapy, attending support groups, or a combination of these treatments… Despite its high treatment success rate, nearly two out of three people suffering with depression do not actively seek nor receive proper treatment."[21]

The combination of medication and psychotherapy (even brief counseling) provides the quickest and most sustained response. In an article titled "Cognitive Behavioral Therapy for Depression Medication," Dr. Jerry L. Halverson says, "Several meta-analyses of studies of the combination of psychotherapy and pharmacotherapy for patients with depression have documented an advantage of the combination treatment compared with either treatment alone."[22] In his article "Depression Treatment & Management," Dr. Halverson says, "Combination therapy has also been associated with significantly higher rates of improvement in depressive symptoms; increased quality of life; and better treatment compliance, especially when treatment is needed for longer than 3 months."[23]

Healthcare professionals treat depression with diet and exercise. Many studies over the last two decades have found exercise is an effective treatment for depression—and some show that aerobic exercise can be as effective as antidepressants in treating mild to moderate depression (and with side effects such as improved health and weight management rather than medication side effects).[24] Other research indicates exercise not only boosts your mood,[25] but also sharpens your memory,[26] alleviates anxiety,[27] helps you sleep better,[28] and increases your creativity.[29] One review of aerobic exercise and major depression recommends that "patients participate in three to five exercise sessions per week, for 30 to 45 minutes per session…Furthermore, the majority of research emphasizes that the exercise regimen should be continued for at least 10 to 16 weeks to achieve the greatest antidepressant effect."[30]

A study of 156 men and women 50 years of age or older concluded that even "a modest exercise program is an effective, robust treatment for patients with major depression" and the benefits were "likely to endure, particularly among those who adopt it as a regular, ongoing life activity."[31] A 2018 meta-analysis of 33 clinical trials including 1,877 participants concluded, "Resistance exercise training [(RET)—e.g., weight lifting] significantly reduced depressive symptoms among adults regardless of health status, total prescribed volume of RET, or significant improvements in strength." The researchers added that RET should be considered "as an alternative and/or adjuvant therapy for depressive symptoms."[32]

Not only does exercise treat depression, but it also may actually prevent it. A 2019 report concluded that "physical activity can reduce the risk of depression…Fifteen minutes of vigorous physical activity or an hour of moderate exercise reduced the risk of depression by 26 percent, and researchers said there also was evidence that a lack of exercise may increase the risk of depression."[33]

What you eat may be as important as how you move when it comes to depression. A 2018 study found that people who follow a heart healthy diet, the Dietary Approaches to Stop Hypertension (DASH) diet, which emphasizes eating fruits and vegetables along with low-fat or nonfat dairy, lean meats, and avoiding foods high in salt and sugar, also have a lower chance of developing depression.[34] Other studies suggest that people who follow a Mediterranean diet, which emphasizes fruits, vegetables, and fish, and limits meat and dairy products, also have lower rates of depression.[35] Even people with moderate to severe depression improved their mood and signs of depression by eating a more healthful diet.[36]

The bottom line is: The majority of people who suffer from depression can become healthier—even highly healthy. You don't have to put up with chronic or disabling depression! But first you need to know if you have it or not. The United States Preventive Services Taskforce (USPSTF) and American Academy of Family Physicians recommend screening for depression for *all* adults older than 18 years, regardless of risk factors, using the Patient Health Questionnaire-2 (PHQ-2) screening instrument:

PHQ-2 SCREENING INSTRUMENT FOR DEPRESSION[37]

Over the past two weeks, how often have you been bothered by any of the following problems?	Not at all	Several days	More than half the days	Nearly every day
Little interest or pleasure in doing things	0	1	2	3
Feeling down, depressed, or hopeless	0	1	2	3

Scoring: A score of three or more is considered a positive result and means you should then take the PHQ-9 (tinyurl.com/y3fbru38) or schedule a visit with your healthcare professional if you screen positive.

Multiple screening tests have been developed to address the confounding factors that make depression screening and diagnosis more challenging later in life. The Geriatric Depression Scale is a questionnaire that screens for depression in older patients without dementia that you can find at tinyurl.com/y3fbru38. Again, you should schedule a visit with your healthcare professional if you screen positive.

One free online app, "Moodpath," checks with you three times a day for 14 days to assess emotional and physical well-being and can help you determine if you have clinical depression. It's at tinyurl.com/y78srnjr.

These depression self-evaluation tools are designed to help you determine if you should see a licensed pastoral or healthcare professional about your feelings. They are screening tests only and should never replace a thorough evaluation by your physician, mental health professional, or pastoral professional. Christian psychiatrists often say mental health is biochemical and may need help through diet and medication, psychological health is emotional and may need help through exercise, fresh air, and counseling, whereas spiritual health needs pastoral care and God. Most folks can benefit from all three.

Finally, if you want to save time, there's a test that will allow you to test for stress, anxiety, and depression at tinyurl.com/zr74tjd. The tools in this essential will help you determine which, if any, S-A-D-nesses you might be wrestling with.

According to Reverend Samuel Rodriguez, president of the National Hispanic Christian Leadership Conference, "Christians struggle with depression and even suicidal thoughts. It does not make you less of a Christian. Just like heart disease or cancer does not dilute our Christianity, neither does mental illness." He further states: "Suffering from mental illness is not a sin. Yet, not addressing it may very well be."[38] At the very least, it's a lost opportunity to improve your health and happiness.

5

HEALTHY RELATIONSHIPS

Vivek Murthy, MD, as the nineteenth US Surgeon General, confronted public health crises such as Zika, opioid addiction, e-cigarette abuse, vaccination refusals, and obesity.[1] Then he sounded a new alarm saying, "It turns out that loneliness is associated with a reduction in your lifespan."[2] He called it a loneliness epidemic in 2017.[3]

The most recent research in 2019 identified "alarmingly high" levels of loneliness that peaks in our mid 50s.[4] Dr. Ellen Lee wrote, "It's linked to poor mental health, substance abuse, cognitive impairment, and worse physical health, including malnutrition, hypertension and disrupted sleep." It can also "increase stress and weaken a person's immune system."[5]

Loneliness is not just epidemic in the US. In 2018, British Prime Minister Theresa May described loneliness as "one of the greatest public health challenges of our time." She appointed a Minister for Loneliness and her government is rolling out a strategy to tackle the issue head-on.[6] In the US, loneliness is also very common. A 2018 study from the American Association of Retired Persons (AARP) Foundation found more than a third of adults over 45 are lonely.[7] A 2019 study from the University of California San Diego School of Medicine reported 76 percent of people had moderate-high loneliness. A UCLA study concluded that loneliness is reaching "epidemic" levels.[8]

Nighttime radio host Delilah writes a chapter in Joe Battaglia's book *Unfriended*, saying, "It seems we are more connected, yet lonelier and more isolated than ever before."[9] Joe adds, "We are wired to have community and smartphones cannot meet our needs for love, acceptance, touch, and connection."[10]

Researchers are increasingly discovering that "loneliness is a common source of distress, suffering, and impaired quality of life in older persons."[11] A group of geriatricians from the University of California at San Francisco wrote, "The concept of loneliness is only starting to be recognized as a separate entity from social isolation and depression."[12] One editorialist, after studying loneliness, concluded, "Simply stated, we are wired for relationships. We need one another and function healthier in relationships."[13]

After studying loneliness, Jessica Olien wrote, "Loneliness is a serious health risk. Studies of elderly people and social isolation concluded that those without adequate social interaction were twice as likely to die prematurely. The increased mortality risk is comparable to that from smoking. And loneliness is about twice as dangerous as obesity. Social isolation impairs immune function and boosts inflammation, which can lead to arthritis, type 2 diabetes, and heart disease. Loneliness is breaking our hearts, but as a culture we rarely talk about it."[14] In fact, loneliness has the same effect as 15 cigarettes a day in terms of negative health outcomes.[15]

Loneliness not only hurts us physically, emotionally, and spiritually, but it can kill. In a meta-analysis of 148 studies and 300,000 participants, researchers concluded that one of the major causes of premature death is loneliness. The results indicated "a 50 percent increased likelihood of survival for participants with stronger social skills." The researchers commented that the 50 percent greater chance of survival (in healthy relationships) is comparable to the "effects of quitting smoking and it exceeds many well-known risk factors for mortality (e.g., obesity, physical inactivity)."[16]

"Dr. John Cacioppo, one of the foremost authorities on loneliness, states that the number of people in your life does not inoculate you from experiencing loneliness. Rather, it's the feeling of being lonely that places the brain and body at risk," writes Gillian Leithman.

"Cacioppo equates feeling lonely with feeling hungry. We compromise our survival and well-being when either is ignored."[17]

A Dutch study examined more than 2,000 men and women aged 65 to 86. Whereas none of the participants had signs of dementia at the outset of the study, results revealed that those who reported loneliness had a 64 percent increase in the risk of developing dementia.[18] Leithman observes, "People also experience an increase in loneliness when they retire from work. That's why you want to make sure you're retiring to something, and that you have friends outside of your place of employment."[19]

Love, social support, intimacy, security, safety, satisfaction, connectedness, and community—these terms all relate to a common theme in the medical literature. When we feel loved, nurtured, appreciated, valued, cared for, and supported, we are much more likely to be happier and healthier. A Harvard study tracked a group of men for almost 80 years. The bottom line was that loving relationships are the key to happiness and health. It was not money or status but strong interpersonal relationships that led to the greatest life satisfaction, whereas those who were isolated had declines in mental and physical health as they aged.[20] In November 2015, Robert Waldinger, the director of the study, shared this key finding in a widely popular Ted Talk that has been viewed close to 14 million times.[21] Clearly there's an appetite for learning what to prioritize to have more fulfilling lives.

Why is this? A number of explanations can be found in research. One study of almost 12,000 individuals examined Japanese men who lived in Japan and compared them to Japanese men who had moved to Hawaii or California. The researchers examined smoking, diet, exercise, cholesterol levels, and social support (the maintenance of social networks and family and community ties). The group with the lowest social support (the California group) had a threefold to fivefold increase in heart disease. The researchers concluded that social networks and close family ties help protect against disease and premature death.[22]

University of Texas researchers evaluated patients who had undergone open-heart surgery. They found those who lacked involvement in organized social groups—a flat relational wheel—had a fourfold increase in the risk of death. Those who reported that they did not draw strength from their religion—a flat spiritual wheel—were three times more likely to die within six months after surgery. These risks were additive, as those who did not engage in organized social activity and who did not draw strength from their religion were more than seven times as likely to die within six months of their surgery.[23]

Other research has shown a strong association between lack of social support and low high-density lipoprotein (HDL) cholesterol levels. HDL cholesterol is the good—or healthy—cholesterol that protects the heart. Lonely people tend to have low HDL cholesterol not explained by diet, physical exercise, alcohol abuse, age, menopause, or smoking. A meta-analysis of more than 1,700 studies concluded that low social support (loneliness) is a risk factor for the development of heart disease in previously healthy individuals, and it also worsens the prognosis of patients with established heart disease.[24]

Many social science researchers are now saying, apart from our genetics, the most powerful across-the-board factor in predicting premature death and disease is lack of social support. Researchers have looked at a variety of relationship measures, such as a sense of being accepted and loved by others and a sense that the support or help of others is available. Almost all these studies conclude that social support affects health positively.[25] People who believe that no one cares for them, who don't feel close to anyone, or who feel they have no one in whom to confide or to help them out of a bind not only have poorer health but are more likely to die prematurely.

In a trailblazing 2010 meta-analysis of 148 studies involving more than 300,000 participants, US researchers revealed that greater social connection was associated with a 50 percent reduced risk of early death.[26] An even larger 2015 review of 70 studies including 3.4 million people reported that, "each risk factor [social isolation, loneliness, living alone] has a significant and equivalent effect on risk for mortality, which exceeds the risk associated with obesity."[27]

Dr. Julianne Holt-Lunstad, Professor of Psychology at Brigham Young University, writes, "Lacking social connection carries a risk that is comparable, and in many cases, exceeds that of other well-accepted risk factors, including smoking up to 15 cigarettes per day, obesity, physical inactivity, and air pollution."[28]

It's important to understand what we do *not* mean by *loneliness*. For example, many people, especially those who have lost a spouse or who are introverts may live by themselves or spend the majority of their time away from the company of others and be perfectly healthy. Reginald Finger, MD, MPH, writes, "As long as one has regular meaningful contact with others who care and value you, you might not suffer loneliness even if living by oneself. On the other hand, a person can feel very much 'alone in a crowd.' Being with all kinds of people in superficial ways all day long can be more toxic in this way than solitude."[29]

Another reason loneliness kills is that a lonely person is more likely to practice unhealthy habits—such as abusing tobacco, alcohol, food, or drugs—but this accounts for only a portion of their risk. Anger, depression, high-stress jobs, low socioeconomic status, and lack of social support often go hand in hand with loneliness. When these risk factors come together in one person, their effects are compounded and can be explosively dangerous to one's health.

One way the government of Great Britain will be helping people overcome loneliness is by implementing a practice called *social prescribing*. By 2023, all doctors in England will be able to "refer patients experiencing loneliness to community activities and voluntary services" as an alternative to prescribing medication. "Such activities could include cooking, dance classes, walking clubs, or art groups, all of which will receive funding from the government and are intended to reduce demand on the NHS [National Health Service] and improve patients' quality of life."[30]

Happy and healthful living requires positive social relationships in family and community. Abundant life is not individual, it's social; it's living with others. Human beings truly live only insofar as they are related to others with whom they share life and love—with whom they serve God, family, and community.

Most people are aware of the need for friends and social support. Contemporary American researcher George Barna writes:

Overall, the research paints a portrait of a nation whose adults keep themselves occupied so they do not have to face significant shortcomings…Many people admit to lacking relational connections and meaning in life. Those two factors are critical to gaining joy and fulfillment in life. The common solution is to keep busy and to stimulate ourselves with a variety of new experiences—that way we are not so likely to feel the pain of those fundamental holes in our life. People have discovered that if they fill the gaps with commitments and excitement, then they're less prone to feel the emptiness of loneliness and aimlessness. Of course, that just prolongs the inner despair that eventually cannot be suppressed any longer.[31]

The good news is that reducing loneliness by developing and enriching friendships will improve your overall health. You don't need a large group of friends. Even one or two close friends with whom you share interests and affection can do the trick. Intentionally involve yourself in a variety of positive and healthy social relationships with people you like and admire—and who are willing and able to care about you and for you. Said another way, "Seek out connection: We all need a tribe!" Or, as the Bible teaches, "Let us not neglect our meeting together, as some people do, but encourage one another" (Hebrews 10:25 NLT).

Jesus set an example for us by making time for His friends (John 15:15). He had three best friends, 12 good friends, and 70 friends. Dr. J. Nick Pitts points out, "The smaller the number, the greater the intimacy. Buddies can bless you, but best friends shape you (Proverbs 27:17). You give time to your friends, but they give you life—an invaluable return on investment."[32]

We highly recommend you invest in relationships with Christian friends—a healthy Christian community. Debra Fileta writes, "The concept of Christian community is such an important part of love, because it's within the context of relationships that we have the opportunity to express and receive love."[33] She suggests ten reasons for why it's critical to be in relationship with other believers:[34]

1. Community challenges you to be more like Jesus (Hebrews 10:24-25).

2. Community meets practical needs (Acts 2:42-47).

3. Community carries you emotionally (Galatians 6:2).

4. Community reveals your gifts and talents (Ecclesiastes 4:9-12).

5. Community opens your eyes to the needs of others (1 Thessalonians 5:14).

6. Community empowers your relationship with God (Proverbs 27:17).

7. Community helps meet our need for love (Proverbs 17:17).

8. Community offers opportunities for confession which leads to healing (James 5:16).

9. Community teaches you to work through conflicts (1 Corinthians 1:10).

10. Community gives you the chance to forgive (1 Peter 4:8-11).

If you are currently lonely, recognize the dangers of prolonged loneliness. If you ignore hunger, you starve. The same is true of our need for belonging. If you feel lonely, reach out to others. Don't wait for your phone or doorbell to ring. It is your responsibility—and privilege—to involve yourself in others' lives.

Start by making a list of your friends—not casual acquaintances, but people who know and love you and with whom you interact on a weekly basis. If your list is short, begin another list of things you can do to be a better friend. Check in every day, at least by text, phone, Skype, or FaceTime, with someone close to you. Think of your relationships as a garden that needs to be tended daily—then do it.

And don't forget that pets can help dispel loneliness. If you don't want to own a pet, follow my friend Cynthia's example and volunteer at an animal shelter on weekends. The big smile I see on her face every time she talks about her work at the shelter leads me to believe that her weekly dose of puppy love is making her more highly healthy.

To continue your journey to becoming a highly healthy person, we hope you will fill some of this chapter's prescriptions for building stronger and healthier relationships. As you do, you will avoid loneliness like the life-threatening plague it is.

6

SPIRITUAL WELL-BEING

The latest medical research continues to support what I have been witnessing in my practice for decades—namely, that a person's *spiritual well-being* has a significant positive impact on his or her relational, emotional, and physical health.[1] But there is a huge difference between what I call *biblical* or *positive spirituality* and an external religion in which people go through the motions of religious duties but lack any personal relationship with God.

The most important element of wellness is seeking, knowing, and pleasing our Creator. If we believe in and trust God, if we make having an intimate relationship with Him a priority, if He controls and empowers our lives and we seek our purpose in His grand design, we will experience wholeness at the deepest level of our being.

Augustine, a fourth-century theologian, wrote in *Confessions*, "O Lord...You have made us for yourself, and our heart is restless until it rests in you."[2] Episcopal Bishop Edmund Lee Browning asks, "What does it take to be happy? I think we are happiest when we know ourselves to be in the service of God, focused on a reality larger than ourselves...it is why we are here."[3]

The good news is this: Though God designed each one of us in His own image, we turned away from that divine design to pursue life after our own image, which has resulted in broken and unhealthy lives. Because of His love for us, God sent His Son, Jesus, to live a perfect, exemplary life and then submit to be tortured and crucified to pay the ransom and redeem us from all our wrongdoing. Through accepting

His sacrifice for our sin and submitting to His lordship, we are able daily to submit ourselves to His will, pursue His design, and trust that His grace of love and forgiveness will work to bring about His good pleasure of equipping us and empowering us to live healthful lives—as He continues producing in and through us spiritual fruit that endures, regardless of our circumstances or the state of our relational, emotional, or physical health.

When we talk about spiritual health, we'll incorporate the terms *biblical* or *true* or *positive spirituality*.[4] In an article for health professionals, I wrote, "Positive spirituality is distinguished from the broader terms (faith, morality, or religion) in that it involves an ever-evolving, authentic, and personal relationship with God that is not bound by race, ethnicity, economic status, or class. This relationship promotes the wellness and welfare of others and of self. It includes the beliefs and values by which an individual lives; and, most importantly, it results in the visible spiritual fruit of love, joy, peace, patience, kindness, goodness, faithfulness, gentleness, and self-control."[5] Most Christians will recognize these as the fruit of the Spirit (Galatians 5:22-23).

Researchers have shown that those who internalize biblical teachings—who frequently pray, apply what the Bible says to their lives, believe they have a close relationship with God, and practice what they preach—have high levels of satisfaction in life, a sense of well-being, and overall happiness. In an article I wrote with four colleagues, partially titled, "Positive Spirituality—The Forgotten Factor," we reviewed the evidence showing that positive spirituality improves wellness as well as psychological and physical health outcomes.[6]

Research indicates these benefits are not as effective when one just goes through the motions of religious tradition. People who merely attend worship services and programs in their religious community tend to experience an *external faith* that is less likely to be associated with positive physical or mental health outcomes. Researchers since the 1960s have told us some people use religion in a self-serving, utilitarian way. "Persons with this orientation," they say, "may find religion useful in a variety of ways—to provide security and solace, sociability and distraction, status and self-justification. The embraced creed is lightly held or else selectively shaped to fit more primary needs. In theological terms the extrinsic type turns to God, but without turning away from self."[7]

Religion, for "extrinsics," according to Dale Matthews, MD, "is a means to obtaining another end—health, security, status, power— even though they may not be consciously aware of their own ulterior motives." In his book *The Faith Factor,* Matthews says those who use their religion for their own purposes "ask not what they can do for their religion, but what their religion can do for them."[8]

As you can imagine, people who rate higher on the true spirituality scales, those with positive spirituality who internalize biblical teachings (compared to those relying on external religion), are more likely to experience physical, emotional, and relational health benefits— substantial benefits. For example, recovery from a major depression has been shown to occur much more rapidly and completely for those with the highest ratings of true spirituality. Lowered blood pressure, better surgical outcomes, less substance abuse, and longer survival have also been noted in the research.[9]

According to researcher George Barna, men and women with a true spirituality say they are most satisfied with their present life (91 percent). This upbeat frame of mind may be related to the fact that they are the least likely to say they are lonely (8 percent), in serious debt (9 percent), or stressed out (16 percent). The percentage who admitted to high levels of stress was less than half that measured among adults connected with extrinsic faiths (33 percent) or those who said they were atheistic or agnostic (42 percent).[10]

This Barna survey of more than three thousand randomly chosen adults in the US found that "although they are slightly less than eight percent of the American adult population, atheists and agnostics possess self-perceptions that clearly stand out from those of citizens who maintain some definable faith preference. The nonfaith segment placed highest among the five groups in claiming to be stressed out (42 percent), concerned about the future (68 percent), and lonely (14 percent). They were least likely to be satisfied with their life (68 percent) and were unconcerned about America's moral state (60 percent)."[11]

We're *not* saying that a personal relationship with God is an insurance policy—a guarantee—against disease. It is not. As one of the pastors who reviewed this book wrote, "Healthy, spiritually grounded people drop dead all the time." We've all lost friends and family—wonderful folks—who died far too young. But the medical research is clear that, in general, the deeper a true spiritual faith, the more likely people are to have a better physical, emotional, and relational health. They are much more likely to cope well with illness and to recover from disease.

If spiritual health is crucial to becoming and staying highly healthy, we should be able to find proof in the medical literature—and there is plenty! In his systematic review *Religion, Spirituality, and Health: The Research and Clinical Implications*, Dr. Harold Koenig of Duke University concludes by writing, "A large volume of research shows that people who are more R/S have better mental and physical health and adapt more quickly to health problems compared to those who are less R/S…The majority of studies report strong relationships between R/S and better health."[12]

We're convinced that God wants us to be as physically and emotionally healthy as possible. In fact, the apostle John wrote, "Dear friend, I pray that you may enjoy good health and that all may go well with you, even as your soul is getting along well" (3 John 1:2). God wants us to enjoy healthy relationships with others. But most of all, He wants us to have a healthy relationship with Him.

The Bible promises, "Blessed are all who fear the LORD, who walk in obedience to him" (Psalm 128:1). The Hebrew word *asre*, translated "blessed," means to experience a heightened state of happiness and joy, implying favorable circumstance and enjoyment, while "fear the Lord" is to reverence Him, to worship Him, to serve Him as the Master and King of our lives. It is to walk in His ways, submissive to His Word.

Jim Denison observes, "Such obedience does not earn God's blessing. To the contrary, it positions us to receive what our Father already wanted to give us. He wants to bless His children. He 'longs to be gracious to you' (Isaiah 30:18)." Denison adds that the Bible "does not qualify what kinds of blessings our Father wants to give us. Some may be material, others emotional, relational, physical, or spiritual. But our Maker knows us better than we know ourselves and knows what is for our best. And he promises us that 'everyone' who reveres Him as Lord is blessed by Him. There are no exceptions or qualifications."[13] As David wrote, "You make known to me the path of life; you will fill me with joy in your presence, with eternal pleasures at your right hand" (Psalm 16:11).

The best way we know to become a highly healthy person is to develop a true spirituality that can result in the most important and enduring form of health and vitality. But, according to Dr. Paul Dybdahl, "While most Americans claim to be Christians, closer inspection reveals that a minority have made a personal commitment to Jesus that remains meaningful in their life today. According to Barna's research, approximately 60 percent of Americans have not made such a personal commitment. That means over 170 million people in North America have yet to commit themselves to God."[14] Are you one of them? If so, you may want to know how you can have a personal relationship with God starting today. I explain this in a web post, "The Most Important Blog I've Ever Written." You can find it at tinyurl.com/y9blalvs. It can be summarized in just 32 words:

- We are sinners and in trouble.
- Jesus is the *only* solution to this trouble.
- We accept His solution by repenting of our sin, asking Him to redeem us, and trusting in Him.

In the meantime, we'd like to offer a brief roadmap to test your spiritual health—a simple self-test designed to help you determine how well you are doing in your personal spiritual journey. Be honest. How true is each characteristic of you?

```
1 = Not at all or never
2 = Not much or rarely
3 = Somewhat or occasionally
4 = Often or usually
5 = Completely or always
```

I maintain an intense respect, awe, humility, and gratitude toward God—in acknowledgment of His superiority and perfection.	
I effectively share the substance of my faith with people who have an interest in it.	
I pray for the needs and future of others.	
My decisions are based on spiritual principles and values.	
My speech and behavior please God.	
When I pray, I both speak and listen to God.	
Worship is not just an event I attend—I live my life as an act of worship to God.	
I am held morally and spiritually accountable by others who know and care for me.	
I give away my time, abilities, and money sacrificially for the benefit of the needy.	
I fight injustice and inequality.	
I strive to live out the Golden Rule—to do to others what I want them to do to me.	
My attitudes, values, and thoughts please God.	

Add up your score. A score of 48 or higher indicates you are likely to be spiritually healthy; a score of 24 or lower indicates you may not be spiritually healthy. If your score is lower than you might expect or want, tip 19, "12 Steps for Spiritual Strength Training," has suggestions of steps you could take, beginning today, to raise your spiritual health quotient.

True, positive, biblical spirituality is the path to spiritual wholeness and overall health. It is a lifelong pursuit. A healthy spirituality is the foundation to the hope, health, and well-being for which we all long. How can we settle for anything less?

7

POSITIVE SELF-IMAGE

According to the Cleveland Clinic, "Self-image is the personal view, or mental picture, we have of ourselves,"[1] Mayo Clinic experts write, "Self-esteem affects virtually every facet of your life. Maintaining a healthy, realistic view of yourself isn't about blowing your own horn. It's about learning to like and respect yourself—faults and all."[2]

Researchers at Syracuse University reported, "Low self-esteem predicts more negative affect, less positive affect, greater stress severity, and greater symptom severity in daily life. There are a number of health benefits to a healthy self-esteem."[3] The Henry Ford Health System says there are six emotional, mental, and physical benefits of a healthy self-esteem:[4]

1. Your expectations are more in line with reality, and as a result, you're less critical of yourself and others.

2. You're better able to handle stress (and avoid the unhealthy side effects that come with it).

3. You're not as likely to battle feelings of worthlessness, guilt, or shame.

4. You can build strong, honest relationships (and are less likely to stay in unhealthy ones).

5. You have greater confidence in your ability to make good decisions.

6. You bounce back more easily when it comes to life's inevitable setbacks.

A positive outlook on life improves quality of life and prolongs its length. Researchers have found solid evidence that looking on the bright side can both reduce the incidence of heart disease and minimize its consequences. Researchers have found positive well-being was associated with nearly a third reduction in coronary disease in a high-risk population with a family history of heart disease, a nearly 50 percent reduction in those with the strongest family history, and a 13 percent reduction in a national sample, independent of all other traditional heart disease risk factors.[5]

Yale scientists in 2018 reported that older people who "carried a gene linked to dementia but also had very positive attitudes about aging were 50 percent less likely to develop the disorder than less positive people." They added, "The results of this study suggest that positive age beliefs, which are modifiable and have been found to reduce stress, can act as a protective factor, even for older individuals at high risk of dementia."[6] Another study found that positivity can reduce anxiety[7] and increase feelings of happiness.[8] It seems clear that a healthy self-image and positive attitude can lead to a healthier body, mind, and relationships.

Through the years, I have cared for many patients who suffered from a poor self-image or outlook on life. Although most don't die from these maladies, they are diseased from them. In fact, they often suffer terribly—physically, mentally, relationally, and spiritually. How do you see yourself? And how do you think your Creator sees you? Do some serious reflection, and write down (and date) your answers to the following questions:

- Do I like myself? Why or why not?
- Do I believe I am worthy of love? Why or why not?
- When I think of God, which reaction do I feel most strongly—comfort or discomfort?
- What do I think God thinks of me? What would He say about me and His feelings for me?
- On what do I base my self-esteem? Is this a good foundation? Why or why not?

Do you see yourself and your future through God's eyes or your own? If the latter, you may be thinking, *I hear* what *you're saying, but I'm just not sure it's true. I don't feel God's love. I don't feel His acceptance. I don't feel unique or special. I don't feel like He sees me—at all.*

If so, we have some tips for you on how to pump up a deflated self-image. If your self-esteem is low, what can you choose to do to increase your likelihood of becoming highly healthy? Throughout the years, I have developed an advice sheet (a prescription of sorts), to help my patients who suffer from a poor self-image. All five items are supported both biblically and scientifically.

1. Place Your Relationship with God at the Center of Your Life

As we discussed earlier, there is significant scientific evidence that a strong faith in, and personal relationship with, God is associated with a large number of positive mental and physical health outcomes. We believe that the underlying truth of our lives is that we were created by a loving God—in the image of this God—and that knowing Him, serving Him, pleasing Him, and worshipping Him will fulfill our primary purpose in life and eternity. In short, we are hardwired to please and to glorify Him in all we think, say, and do. We have more on this topic in tip 19.

John Piper, in his book *Don't Waste Your Life*, writes:

> The really wonderful moments of joy in this world are not the moments of self-satisfaction, but self-forgetfulness. Standing on the edge of the Grand Canyon and contemplating your own greatness is pathological. At such moments we are made for a magnificent joy that comes from outside ourselves…God created me—and you—to live with a single, all-embracing, all-transforming passion—namely, a passion to glorify God by enjoying and displaying his supreme excellence in all the spheres of life.[9]

2. Read, Memorize, and Meditate on Bible Passages Daily

For years I have given my patients an assignment to memorize and meditate on portions of the Bible relevant to a health issue with which they are wrestling. Several studies have shown that people who spend time reading and reflecting on the Bible daily have better health outcomes. One researcher examined the relationship between Bible study and a healthy marriage and concluded, "There was a fairly strong relationship between both prayer and Bible reading and marital adjustment," and, "A strong commitment to religious practice and ideals can enhance marital stability."[10] Other studies have found that daily Bible reading was associated with greater life satisfaction[11] and greater degrees of hopefulness.[12] Bible reading also may be associated with a protection against alcoholism[13] and depressive symptoms,[14] as well as improve many other mental and physical health measures.[15]

Astonishingly, one's whole way of thinking can be renewed. In fact, the Bible tells us: "Do not conform to the pattern of this world but be transformed by the renewing of your mind" (Romans 12:2). A poor self-image can be transformed into positive self-esteem as we discover how much God loves us and how passionately He wants our lives to be full and meaningful. The renewing of our minds is a gradual process, and it can be enhanced by reading, memorizing, and meditating on the Bible. We have more on this topic in tip 21.

3. Spend Time in Meditation and Prayer Daily

Prayer and times of solitude are high priorities in the lives of highly healthy people. Prayer is simply conversing with God. Meditation is purposefully concentrating and listening with our spiritual ears to what God has already said in Scripture and what His Spirit communicates to our spirits during our conversation with Him. I've written an article reviewing the many medical studies that have shown the significant effects of prayer you can find at tinyurl.com/y7fkbt54.

Studies have also shown a positive correlation between activities such as prayer and Bible reading and satisfaction in life.[16] Researchers believe time spent in meditation and prayer—especially when joined with Bible study—takes a person's focus away from a potentially pathological concentration on self—a focus that not only lowers self-esteem but also reduces life satisfaction and well-being. By concentrating on ourselves and our problems, while failing to see the bigger picture, we can contribute to our own demise. Investing as little as five to ten minutes a day in meditation and prayer can change you. If you've never considered investing time in yourself, now is the time to start. Set your alarm clock fifteen minutes earlier. Get out of bed and enjoy the luxury of time alone—for you and with your Creator. We have more on this topic in tip 22.

4. Avoid Negative Self-Talk

Being overly critical of ourselves—regularly beating ourselves up—makes for low self-esteem. People can improve their moods, their attitudes, and their overall health by changing the way they think and the things they tell themselves about themselves, life, and God. What we think is what we declare to ourselves in the privacy of our own minds. One large review concluded that while an optimistic attitude does wonders for patients' recovery, negative attitudes and critical self-talk decrease one's likelihood of becoming highly healthy.[17]

The apostle Paul wrote, "Whatever is true, whatever is noble, whatever is right, whatever is pure, whatever is lovely, whatever is admirable—if anything is excellent or praiseworthy—think about such things. Whatever you have learned or received or heard from me or seen in me—put it into practice. And the God of peace will be with you" (Philippians 4:8-9). What we think and how we think—and how we talk to ourselves about what we think—has a direct impact on our peace of mind. The type of thinking Paul has in mind improves our moods, our immune functions, and our health.

We cannot overemphasize the importance of these first four steps. Neuroscientists have developed stunning brain scanning technologies, showing how our emotions and thoughts actually can change our brain structure. "Scientists now affirm that how and where we focus our attention dictates the content of the brain structure we create," writes author Kitty Crenshaw and clinical psychologist Cathy Snapp, PhD. "By choosing to focus our attention (mindfulness and prayer) on uplifting emotional content (positivity and hope) and sustain that moment for 25 seconds (installation), we little by little change our brain structure, which changes mental activity, which changes bio-chemical communication in the body, which genetically changes gene expression and thus our physical, mental, and emotional well-being."[18] We have more on this topic in tip 22.

5. Serve Others

People who have healthy self-esteem are not self-absorbed. Being comfortable in our own skin empowers us to serve and truly give of ourselves to others—just the way Jesus commanded us. Loving our neighbors as ourselves is a virtue of the highest order. Yet those who practice this discipline will always testify, "You get more than you give." People who make serving others a high priority have the greatest like-lihood of becoming highly healthy.

Steve Wilson, a psychologist and self-proclaimed "joyologist," says, "There is a kind of unhappiness that cannot be repaired by getting, because it requires giving. There is a kind of dissatisfaction, disappoint-ment, and absence of joy that is remedied by giving something out, doing something for others…Happiness is an inside job that consists of…remembering who you are (precious), finding your source, laugh-ing often, serving with love."[19]

Researchers studied 2,153 older men in Japan and found a fasci-nating pattern. Self-reported health status among men tended to be higher among those who helped other people—and the more these men helped others, the better their health. Those who were more involved in helping others (and had a higher degree of health) were also the men who engaged in private religious practices.[20] We encourage you to find specific ways you can make serving other people a higher priority. What will you do differently in the month ahead to become healthier in this area?

Think about a place in your community or church where you can serve. Commit to serving at a food pantry, a homeless shelter, a hospi-tal, a senior citizen center, the humane society. There are hundreds of other options. Pick one—any one. But choose a place and a time to give of your time and talent to others less fortunate.

"A simple step is to begin the process of helping others is by doing

Acts of Random Kindness (ARK) events," writes Thomas McKnight, MD, MPH. "What my daughter and I do, when in my truck doing errands or driving around, is look for simple ways to help someone else, like loading groceries for an elderly person at Walmart. This increases the release of the 'feel good' brain hormone dopamine."[21] We have more on this topic in tips 1 and 2.

So, in conclusion, we ask you: How is your view of yourself? When you look at yourself in the mirror or think about how you've lived your life, do you feel positive or negative? Do you feel healthy or unhealthy?

Highly healthy people almost always have a positive view of themselves. We're not saying they are conceited—or that their egos are over-inflated—but that they've come to accept themselves, warts and all, and respect themselves. If you suffer from a deflated self-image, it's time to take another look in the mirror. See yourself as God sees you. He designed and created the person you see reflected there.

The key to a realistic and positive self-image is agreeing with God about ourselves. Henri Nouwen writes of how God would speak to you:

> I have called you by name, from the very beginning. You are mine and I am yours. You are my Beloved, on you my favor rests. I have molded you in the depths of the earth and knitted you together in your mother's womb. I have carved you in the palms of my hands and hidden you in the shadow of my embrace. I look at you with infinite tenderness and care for you with a care more intimate than that of a mother for her child. I have counted every hair on your head and guided you at every step. Wherever you go, I go with you, and wherever you rest, I keep watch. I will give you food that will satisfy all your hunger and drink that will quench all your thirst. I will not hide my face from you. You know me as your own as I know you as my own. You belong to me. I am your father, your mother, your brother, your sister, your lover and your spouse…Wherever you are I will be. Nothing will ever separate us. We are one.[22]

You were designed to have a life that is meaningful and infused with a sense of well-being. God designed you to experience and dispense love (rather than loathing), joy (rather than sorrow), peace (rather than distress), patience (rather than pigheadedness), kindness (rather than meanness), goodness (rather than hostility), faithfulness (rather than disloyalty), gentleness (rather than callousness), and self-control (rather than instability) (see Galatians 5:22-23).

By seeing yourself as your Creator sees you and learning to incorporate His plan and design into how you live and what you do, you will become empowered to live out God's purpose for your life. We believe that your Creator has designed you for a specific purpose—and being true to that purpose will result in genuine and lasting joy and satisfaction. Research has shown that only about 25 percent of Americans have a clear sense of purpose[23]—and having purpose is linked to better sleep quality,[24] reduced all-cause mortality and cardiovascular events such as fewer strokes and heart attacks,[25] improved cognitive function and reduced risk of Alzheimer's,[26] and a lower risk of premature death.[27]

Regardless of your past—broken dreams, failed relationships, etc.—the almighty God, who loves you, has a plan for your life. Seek His face, embrace His love, and don't stop until His plan for your life is your plan for your life. Nothing else could be more important. As Jesus said, "A thief is only there to steal and kill and destroy. I came so they can have real and eternal life, more and better life than they ever dreamed of" (John 10:10 MSG).

8

UNCOVER YOUR PASSION

I n my 40-plus years as a physician, I've met many who have waited until the twilight of their lives to begin living their dreams by finally realizing their purpose—their passion or destiny—and discover the healing power of following their God-given hopes and vision. They find freedom in *not* obeying the unrighteous or unbiblical dictates, expectations, and preferences of others. These highly healthy people begin to discover, develop, nurture, and nourish the path in life that God designed them to walk—a path that will always result in satisfaction and blessing.

Living by Design

We believe each of us was meticulously created by the Master Designer—God Himself. We exist for a reason, and we are loved by our Creator beyond our wildest imaginings. We are designed for a purpose. Jesus stated that He came to earth so that each of us "may have life and have it to the full" (John 10:10).

In writing about the beautiful benefits of a personal relationship with God, Christian psychiatrists Frank Minirth and Paul Meier observe, "The believer has an opportunity to find meaning and purpose in his or her life." They continue, "For believers, purpose and meaning in life is recognizing that we are not our own, but instead we belong to [God]." They ask each of us this question: "Have you dedicated your life to Him for whatever He wills?" If you have, "You will then discover your calling and internal identity as God's servant and ambassador and look for ever-increasing opportunities that will allow you the most freedom in expressing who you are for the glory of God."[1]

In a letter to the Christians in Rome, the apostle Paul wrote, "I urge you, brothers and sisters, in view of God's mercy, to offer your bodies as a living sacrifice, holy and pleasing to God—this is your true and proper worship. Do not conform to the pattern of this world but be transformed by the renewing of your mind" (Romans 12:1-2).

The Greek word *syschēmatizomai*, translated as "conform," means to be molded by external forces. The word for "world," *aiōn*, refers to the world system or values that is opposed to biblical teaching. So, as followers of Jesus, we are not to be pressured into or pushed along by unbiblical beliefs.

Then the Greek word *metamorphoomai* (the root for our word *metamorphosis*), translated as "transformed," means to be changed from the inside out. Paul is calling believers to a radical change at the deepest level of their hearts and minds—to be transformed into people who live out a genuinely biblical worldview.

Jesus said, "Seek first [God's] kingdom and his righteousness, and all these things will be given to you as well" (Matthew 6:33). By *these things*, He was referring to food and clothing—the necessities of life. If we want our lives to be infused with satisfaction, meaning, purpose, hope, and joy, the Bible tells us that it can only happen by knowing God personally and choosing to serve and please Him daily. In contrast, choosing to live outside of the purpose for which we were created inevitably results in a lack of wholeness, a shortage of passion, a deficiency of blessedness, and dissatisfaction—put simply, it results in *disease*. For example, choosing to eat the wrong thing could cause death. Just ask Adam and Eve (Genesis 3:6).

The treatment of this type of dis-ease has two components. The first element we've already talked about is coming to know God and developing a vibrant personal relationship with Him. The second involves living out our God-given hopes and dreams in the context of our Creator's purpose for our lives.

In his book *The Power of Purpose*, Richard Leider points out, "Purpose is not a thing. It is never a static condition we can preserve. Purpose is a continuous activity, questions we ask over and over again. It's a process we live every day. It's a process for listening and shaping our life stories."[2] Not only is finding your life story a key to achieving a high degree of health, but also discovering your role in God's story is critical as well. (For more on this, we recommend Kurt Bruner's book *The Divine Drama: Discovering Your Part in God's Story.*[3])

We have found it challenging to work with patients, students, and colleagues who claim to have a personal relationship with God and yet who still wonder, *What is my purpose? Why am I here? Where is true joy and satisfaction?* Most of these men and women believe that God created them and loves them, yet they sense that they haven't uncovered God's plan for their lives—that they're not in the center of His will. Most of these folks seem to feel there's more to life than they're experiencing. They wish they could be doing something else. Most don't feel significant or fulfilled. They are not at ease, they aren't whole, and aren't experiencing blessedness—they are dis-eased.

What do we prescribe for those who are in this quandary? Three simple words: *Uncover your passion.* Begin the process of determining God's personal plan for your life and act to live it with gusto. How? We prescribe studying the book *Discover Your Destiny* by Bill and Kathy Peel.[4]

I've noticed, though, that most people have an inborn wariness of their own hopes and dreams, It's as though they believe their Creator could not possibly want them to see their dreams come true. Like some of the folks we talked about in the last chapter, they simply do not see themselves as God sees them. And as a result, by not pursuing their hopes and dreams, they forfeit many of the blessings and the deep fulfillment He longs to give them. Mark Batterson wrote a book titled *Chase the Lion: If Your Dream Doesn't Scare You, It's Too Small.* It goes much deeper into this concept.[5]

Take a Look in the Mirror

Before you read any further, take time to consider the following:

- Do I believe God created me uniquely and has a plan for my life?
- Do I believe I'm in the center of God's plan for my life?
- Do I experience joy and satisfaction in my life and work?
- Do I have a sense of partnering with God to bring Him glory and to serve others?

Write out answers to these questions and any others that may come to mind in your journal. Don't be concerned if it takes you a while. It may raise some uncomfortable issues. You don't need to understand everything about God's plan right now—just write down what God brings to mind. Then think, meditate, and pray about what you think God is calling you to do and be.

Finding your God-given passion—living out the hopes and dreams God provides—is becoming what your Creator created you to become. God doesn't want you to be miserable! Rather, He wants you to experience joy and peace as you do the things He created you to accomplish (Ephesians 2:10). Many people think seeking God's will and inflating their spiritual wheel will require them to give up all their dreams and pleasures. In fact, nothing could be unhealthier—or more unbiblical!

Men and women who live their lives strictly in accordance with their own selfish desires are not becoming highly healthy people. Those who seek God's assistance in fulfilling their own agendas will not find their true purpose or enjoy high degrees of health. Even those who do what they were created to do but do it for selfish reasons—for their own benefit and glory—also cannot become highly healthy people who experience lasting satisfaction. It is only those who do what they were created to do—in a right relationship with their Creator and with the right motives (to glorify and please God while serving Him and others)—who have the opportunity to become highly healthy.

How can you discover your destiny—your Creator's purpose for you? How do you get in touch with your God-given hopes and dreams—perhaps abandoned somewhere along life's path—and nurture them back to life? The first step is to recognize, name, and then follow your personal and God-created passion. *Passion* is doing something not just because you like doing it but because it will make a difference in the world in the longer term. Frederick Buechner said, "The place God calls you to is the place where your deep gladness and the world's deep hunger meet." Just doing what you like because it provides personal satisfaction will eventually become dull. There are only so many ways in which you can get satisfaction doing something for yourself.

"*Passion* is such a powerful word, especially in light of its root origin related to suffering as in 'the passion of Christ' and the 'paschal lamb,'" writes family physician Patricia Landry. "When I've been asked what I am 'passionate' about, I stop and think about what is so important to me that I am willing to suffer for it."[6]

With passion, there is no limit to the number of ways in which satisfaction will come to you. Your God-created passion is not simply something you do; it's something you can't not do and something for which you're willing to both sacrifice and suffer.

Uncover Your Passion

We define *passion* as a God-given, deep-seated longing for something—a divinely directed capacity to feel so deeply attracted to doing something that it becomes a source of power and momentum. This type of passion is a persistent and powerful guide toward our God-ordained destiny. It can be suppressed, but it takes energy—and suppressing it causes harm. Because a life-directing passion is placed in each person by God, failing to move toward fulfilling this inner desire can only result in dissatisfaction, discontentment, disappointment, and displeasure.

Thomas Edison wrote, "If we all did the things we are capable of doing, we would literally astound ourselves."[7] We'd alter his words a bit to say, "If we all did what we were called by God to do, we would live astounding lives!"

Take time to list your passions in your journal. What do you long to do? What are your deepest desires? Write down the things you perceive are keeping you from following your God-given passion. List every obstacle you can imagine. What would it take to follow your passion? What support do you have? What would you need now and along the way? Helen Keller, who overcame blindness and deafness, wrote, "Life is either a daring adventure or nothing."[8] No matter your age, it is never too late to become the person you were designed to be.

Having trouble finding your passion, your direction in life? Consider taking a walk and spending time alone with your Creator. Ponder some of the principles we've discussed. Then, in a day or so, reread this chapter, slowly. Here's why: If you don't get this idea, you won't get the ideas that will follow, and it will be difficult for you to become a highly healthy person.

Don't expect this chapter to make perfect sense—at least not right away. Let this information seep into your soul. Meditate on it and pray about it. Why? Because a passionate sense of purpose and personal destiny is the foundation to higher levels of health. "Passion," says psychiatrist Boyd J. Slomoff, "is what can change choice into commitment. It is a guarantee of reward that is as everlasting as your participation."[9]

We've now completed 80 percent of our reflections on the ten essentials of highly healthy people. We know the journey hasn't been easy. But the truth is, no reward worth seeking and having is easy to obtain.

Most of what we've covered has involved you working with, and on, yourself. Now we're going to shift gears a bit. Although there is much you can do to improve your personal health, it should be obvious that you also need the expertise of healthcare professionals—a winning healthcare team. In the next two chapters, we'll address how you can customize your healthcare plan by becoming your own quarterback and teaming up with the best health professionals you can find.

9

PERSONAL RESPONSIBILITY

Many of my patients tell me they feel baffled, even powerless, in the face of myriad healthcare options. They also seem confused over medical reporting in the media. As one patient told me, "One day they say a high-protein diet is healthy—and the next day they say it's deadly. Who should I believe? Can't you doctors ever get the story straight?"

The issue is not just the doctors. The issue also involves the patient. As long as healthcare consumers depend completely on others—even educated professionals—who have differing opinions about everything from aloe to zinc, from acupressure to Zen, from Pap smears to cancer treatments—they are likely to become more, not less, confused.

It is no wonder. A tidal wave of medical information hits us every day—from our morning paper and the national magazines to the evening news, TV magazine shows, and radio reports—plus the massive amounts of information available on the internet. Many times, consumers have reports on medical studies days or even weeks before the medical journals get to doctors' offices. And the headlines seldom accurately convey the science.

"I don't know if you're a football fan," I told a patient recently, "but let me give you an analogy I've shared with my patients for years: You need to become your own healthcare quarterback. You'll need a good primary care physician as your coach—someone who's a medical expert and willing to listen to you, to coach and advise you— sometimes even to fuss at you and push you. You may also need some specialists—assistant coaches. These coaches are trained in a specific aspect of the game. They know almost everything there is to know about the part of the body they're in charge of, but they can't see the entire game in the same way you and your coach can. The best teams— the ones that win the most—have great quarterbacks working with great coaches. When it comes to your health, you need to learn how to call the plays. *You* must take charge of your healthcare and become your own healthcare quarterback."

A reviewer of this chapter wrote me the following note:

> I'm not qualified to sort through all the options myself and make a sound medical decision. I need an expert to inform me about the whole process and recommend the best treatment options. This is the doctor's job, as far as I'm concerned.

We totally agree! That's exactly what your doctor should do as your healthcare coach—make recommendations and explain in clear terms the nature of your medical problem and your treatment options. The doctor should advise you on what is normally the best plan for your particular medical problem. Note, though, the words *recommendations* and *options*. Your doctor needs to give you the information you need and let you make the final decision on what play to call.

As you learn how to become your own healthcare quarterback, we encourage you to do at least two things: First, be proactive and take more responsibility than you have taken in the past. Dr. Rosenfeld points out, "Knowledge is power. You should have as much information as possible about your condition—and your rights—so that you have the confidence to share in the decisions that affect your health, the quality of your life, and survival itself. The better prepared you are to ask informed questions, the better your chances of receiving optimum medical care."[1]

Second, find a primary care physician (PCP) to be your healthcare coach. You *don't* want a healthcare coach who will overwhelm you with data, research conclusions, and divergent opinions—and then leave you with too much information to process. Look for a physician who will guide you in exploring the best options regarding your healthcare and treatment, then recommend your best options—but will let you make your choice.

We are not saying that you must become a medical expert to have any hope of becoming highly healthy—of course not! We are saying that when you actively participate in your care—in partnership with a physician who encourages such teamwork—you are operating according to the best model of medicine, the one most likely to result in your becoming highly healthy. That is why finding a terrific healthcare coach to inform and guide you should be your first move.*

How to Take Charge of Your Healthcare

To anyone who wants to work successfully with their healthcare professionals to make medically reliable and biblically sound choices about their health, I recommend my GUEST acrostic[2] to increase your skills as a healthcare quarterback:

G: Get the facts
U: Understand the layers of healthcare
E: Explore all treatment options
S: Seek wise spiritual counsel
T: Take a personal inventory

G: Get the Facts

Always begin your journey to health by asking your healthcare professional for a thorough summary of the issue at hand. Here are several questions to ask:

- What is my diagnosis?

---

* A word of caution to our brothers and sisters who are healthcare professionals: You cannot be both the *quarterback* and the *coach* for yourself. Sir William Osler, often called the *Father of Modern Medicine* and one of the four founding professors of Johns Hopkins Hospital famously wrote, "A physician who treats himself has a fool for a patient." (Sir William Osler, in Robert Bennet Bean and William Bennett Bean, *Sir William Osler: Aphorisms from His Bedside Teachings and Writings* (Springfield, IL, Charles C. Thomas Publishers, 1961), 54. Michael Dorman added, "He who doctors himself has a fool for a physician." Michael Dorman, *King of the Courtroom: Percy Foreman for the Defense* (New York: Delacorte Press, 1969), 58.

- How certain are you that this diagnosis is correct?

- Could this be any other disease or condition besides the one being considered?

- What are the causes of my condition?

- What other symptoms might be seen?

- What tests or assessments are recommended? What will they cost? Will they be covered by insurance?

- Where can I learn more about this disorder? Are there any internet sites you recommend? Are there any resources you would recommend? Do you have any patient-education materials you could give me?

- Do you have other patients with the same condition who can contact me and share what they've learned and experienced?

If your appointment time with your healthcare professional is too short, reschedule a longer appointment to discuss your concerns. Bring a list of all your questions. Also consider bringing your spouse or a trusted friend to listen, take notes, and ask questions. If your health-care professional can't or won't spend the time with you that you desire, seek the opinion of one who will. This is your right and responsibility. For recommended tests or referrals, call your insurance company if you are unsure about what's covered.

Double-check everything you hear and learn. If it's true, you'll be able to find documentation from several sources. If the sources conflict, ask your physician to help you sort out the contradictions. Don't hesitate to request (even insist upon) a second opinion when the disease or treatment plan is controversial, uncertain, or can be life- or body-changing. And, if those two opinions differ, seek a third opinion. Your emphasis should be on gathering useful and reliable information. It's your job to become educated about your disease or disorder.

U: Understand the Different Layers of Healthcare

You can gain care and information from several levels of the healthcare system.

PRIMARY CARE

The first and most basic level of medical care is primary care. Family physicians, pediatricians, general (or primary care) internists, and geriatricians provide this care. Many primary care physicians have midlevel professionals or physician extenders working alongside them. Physician assistants (PA), certified nurse midwifes, and nurse practitioners can all help provide primary care and assist you in coordinating any specialists, tests, or procedures you might need. PCPs are generalists who are trained to diagnose and treat more than 90 percent of the problems you have.

Joel E. Yeager, MD, writes, "US adults who have a primary care physician have 33 percent lower health care costs and 19 percent lower odds of dying than those who see only a specialist. As a nation, we would save $67 billion each year if everybody used a primary care provider as their usual source of care."[3] A 2019 study published in *JAMA Internal Medicine* found parts of the US with more PCPs had lower mortality rates and increased life expectancy than those with fewer doctors.[4]

For most patients, the best choice for a healthcare coach and advocate will be a primary care professional. You'll be the quarterback of your healthcare team. You call the plays. But your coach will be your PCP.

SECONDARY CARE

Secondary-care physicians are also called *specialists*. They may care for acute conditions that cannot be treated in an outpatient setting due to the severity of illness, such as emergency or urgent care professionals. They may care for a single organ system or gender. For example, neurologists care for problems of the brain, spinal cord, and nerves, while obstetrician-gynecologists care for women's problems. Specialists are highly trained to care for problems, but only in their area of expertise. For some patients, because of their health problem, their best choice for a healthcare coach or advocate is a specialist. Examples might include a cancer patient's oncologist, a heart patient's cardiologist, or a senior citizen's geriatrician.

TERTIARY CARE

For those problems that occur rarely, or for treatments that are new, a patient is best treated in the large medical centers usually associated with medical schools, research centers, or residency training programs. These centers care for the sickest of the sick. Whereas a primary care physician might see one case of a particular disease in years of practice, a tertiary care physician may treat many each year. They often conduct research and are usually up to date with the newest treatments, as well as experimental treatments.

QUATERNARY CARE

This care is even more specialized. It's usually provided in what is called a *Center of Excellence*. Verywellhealth.com contributor Trisha Torrey says, "Because it is so specific, not every hospital or medical center offers quaternary care…The types of care that might be considered to be quaternary would be experimental medicine and procedures as well as highly uncommon and specialized surgeries."[5]

E: Explore Treatment Options

Whenever possible, obtain complete information on the risks, benefits, and costs of each treatment option. Ask every healthcare expert you see, "What are *all* the potential treatments available to me, and how do you suggest we analyze them to come up with my best treatment option?"

Ask how your condition can be expected to progress with treatment—and without treatment. Even for the most commonly recommended options, ask the professional, "Will you discuss with me *all* the possible risks and benefits of what you are recommending? What will they cost? Of these costs, how much will I need to pay?"

Some healthcare professionals aren't used to caring for people who are their own healthcare quarterbacks. Some may seem bothered by these kinds of discussions. If your doctor seems bothered or distracted, consider saying, "Doctor [or therapist or spiritual counselor], you seem distracted [busy, bothered]. Would there be a better time to schedule with you to discuss my concerns?"

When one of my friends asked a question like this of her doctor, she was told, "I'm not sure I have the time for this type of thing."

"No problem," she calmly replied. "Can you suggest another doctor who does?"

Her doctor smiled. He got the point. From then on, he made the time for her. But if he hadn't, she was prepared to go elsewhere to obtain the healthcare information she needed.

Phil once asked several questions of a urologist who was treating him. The urologist replied, "I don't have time for your questions." That was Phil's last visit with him.

S: Seek Wise Spiritual Counsel

Spiritual guidance and counsel, especially if you're facing a life-threatening situation, is a critical component of your healthcare. The Bible teaches, "Is anyone among you sick? Let them call the elders of the church to pray over them and anoint them with oil in the name of the Lord. And the prayer offered in faith will make the sick person well; the Lord will raise them up. If they have sinned, they will be forgiven" (James 5:14-15).

Pastors, priests, elders, deacons, and other spiritual professionals such as parish nurses, Christian counselors, and pastoral counselors are also obvious selections for spiritual care. If you are not active in a faith community but desire spiritual guidance, consider calling your local hospital to see if there's a chaplain on staff. Hospital chaplains are delighted to assist you as you seek wisdom and comfort in the midst of a medical dilemma or crisis. In addition, in most communities, Christian lay ministers are trained by the Order of St. Luke[6] or the Stephen Ministries[7] to minister to the spiritual health needs of others.

They may ask you challenging questions about your spiritual health. They are often able to give you wise counsel and certainly will be able to pray with and for you. They may also be able to put you in contact with others who have wrestled with the same problems.

T: Take a Personal Inventory

Begin a personal inventory—in writing—about your healthcare needs. Take quiet time to think, meditate, pray, and journal. Don't just record the facts you're discovering. Record what others are telling you as well. Record how you feel about your medical, emotional, relational, and spiritual challenges. Be honest. This journal is for no one's eyes but yours.

As part of your inventory, consider what your own intuition is telling you about your medical problems. If you had no fear of any consequences, what would you do? If money were no object, what would you do? What do you sense God is leading you to do or not do?

Write out your prayers and spend plenty of time listening to the answers that come to you through your own spiritual ears, through the wise guidance of others, and through the circumstances that unfold. Record all answers that emerge from your time of prayer.

Finally, write about the support you feel you need, both now and throughout your treatment. What support is already available to you? How can you find the support you need?

Make Well-Informed Decisions

Following the GUEST steps can assist you in making wise healthcare decisions that are fully informed, spiritually sound, and satisfying. But remember, after all the learning and prayer and reflection, your final decision will involve a step of faith.

It's important to add a caveat. Patients sometimes think that following this process somehow guarantees good results. It does not, but it can distinctly improve your chances for the best possible outcome.

10

YOUR HEALTHCARE TEAM

Being highly healthy requires not only that you take personal responsibility for your healthcare and choose to be your own healthcare quarterback (essential 9), but also that you wisely choose your healthcare team, which should be made up of a healthcare coach (your primary care physician) and other healthcare professionals you may need (your team players). Once you've become convinced of the value of healthcare that embraces the physical, emotional, relational, and spiritual aspects of who you were created to be, you can begin to build a winning healthcare team that shares, or is able to support, your beliefs and philosophy.

Pharmacist

A critical part of your healthcare team, especially if you take prescription medications, nonprescription medications, or natural medications (herbs, vitamins, or supplements) is a trusted pharmacist. Most pharmacies have consultation areas where you can visit with a pharmacist. If you are taking more than one medication (prescription or nonprescription drugs, including herbs, vitamins, or supplements), we recommend reviewing these with a pharmacist. This is especially true if you are seeing multiple specialists who may not be aware of possible drug interactions that come with medications your other doctors give you, because they are unaware of those medications or don't use them often.

Dental Health Professionals

Your dentist and dental hygienist can have a positive influence on your physical, emotional, and relational health. The connection between oral health and overall health is clear in multiple studies. As one insurance company writes, "From heart disease to diabetes and oral cancer to premature births, dental care has an impact on total health and well-being."[1]

Mental Health Professionals

Psychologists, professional counselors, social workers, and marriage and family therapists are licensed, certified, and trained to provide diagnosis and therapy for a variety of mental, emotional, and relational problems. You can call the counseling department at Focus on the Family (1-800-A-FAMILY) to find competent faith-based counselors in your area.

Psychiatrists are physicians (MD or DO) specially trained in evaluating and treating mental health and disease. They prescribe medications, order laboratory and other diagnostic tests, and admit patients to the hospital when necessary. Psychiatrists usually work with a team of mental health professionals.

Registered Dietitian Nutritionist (RDN)

RDNs are an invaluable source regarding nutrition and dietary management of a host of conditions. Many have private practices; others serve on the staff of local hospitals and are available for private consultations. Your nutrition affects your physical, emotional, and relational health. If you think your or your family's dietary habits need repair, a dietitian will be able to suggest healthy strategies for improving your nutritional health.

Chiropractors

Many people include a chiropractor on their healthcare team. These professionals utilize musculoskeletal therapies. Chiropractic care has evolved into two schools of thought: (1) the *isolationists*, who believe their therapy can prevent and treat most diseases without the assistance of other healthcare professionals, often trying to convince patients to sign long-term care arrangements, and (2) the *science-based rationalists*, who desire to be part of a traditional healthcare team. Chiropractor Samuel Homola writes, "Science-based chiropractors make appropriate judgments about the nature of their patients' problems, determine whether these problems lie within their scope, and make appropriate referrals for problems that do not. If you can find one who uses manipulation and physical therapy appropriately and who is willing to coordinate with your personal physician, you can benefit from the best that both have to offer."[2]

Alternative Healthcare Professionals

More and more Americans are inviting alternative, or complementary, healthcare professionals to join their healthcare team. Many of these alternative practitioners are unlicensed and unregulated, particularly those who deal in alternative nutritional therapy. In *Alternative Medicine: The Christian Handbook*,[3] Dónal O'Mathúna, PhD, and I wrote about the most popular alternative therapies, herbal remedies, vitamins, and dietary supplements—everything from acupuncture to yoga and aloe to zinc. We describe several alternatives to traditional care that have evidence to support their use—and other alternatives with good evidence that they could complement traditional medicine. However, we also describe many alternative therapies that have little or no evidence to back up their claims, and we found some to be dangerous. We concluded that if you choose to add alternative therapies to your healthcare, or if you seek the services of an alternative practitioner, do so under the supervision of your healthcare coach—your primary care physician.

Faith Community and Prayer Partners

Socialization is good for your health, but socialization in a Christian community is *exceptionally* good for your health. One of the keys to becoming highly healthy is having people who will pray with you and for you. Increasingly, studies show that prayer affects many health outcomes, including anxiety disorders, cardiovascular disease, depression, disabilities, marital satisfaction, pain relief, recovery from heart attack and surgery, an intensive care unit stay, substance abuse, and generalized well-being. One research group demonstrated the "strongest factors for well-being (life satisfaction and happiness) were frequency of prayer and prayer experience." They also found that conversational and meditative prayers were more strongly related to well-being than ritual or rote prayer.[4]

If you are not a person of prayer, find someone who is. Ask this person if they will begin to pray for you and teach you to pray. If you don't regularly read and study the Bible, begin now. Find a friend or pastor who studies the Bible and ask them to teach you how. Begin reading the Bible every day. Gradually increase your reading time. Ask a bookstore sales associate to help you find a Bible that can provide guidance and interpretation as you read. Both talking with God (prayer) and listening to God (prayer and Bible reading) increase your likelihood of becoming and remaining a highly healthy person.

Support Group

If you're dealing with a chronic health issue, then you'll also benefit from finding a support group—an established group of folks who wrestle with the same health issues with which you struggle. You can locate such groups through local hospitals, national associations, or faith communities. Such groups provide a great forum for the dissemination of useful information and sharing personal experience. They are also helpful to prevent, or treat, isolation, alienation, and loneliness.

The internet has transformed the meaning of the support group concept. Through social media you can find hundreds of groups dealing with the same health issues and decisions as you. But an internet support group can never provide the same level of personal support and healing as people you meet face-to-face. Studies have shown that the majority of medical advice given in internet chat rooms, bulletin boards, or support group websites is inaccurate and sometimes even dangerous.[5] Also, it's not unusual for folks on these sites to try to sell you on scams, schemes, or fraudulent supplements or supplies, while others are in multilevel marketing organizations. Be careful.

Family and Friends

Not only can a friend or family member be a part of your healthcare team, they can often play a critical role. Studies show family and friends are consistently rated as the most vital supports for people with health issues. Studies also have found "patients often believe the presence of a family member leads to an atmosphere of greater empathy and compassion from the professional health care team."[6] The American Academy of Family Physicians points out, "Involvement of family members in the care of the patient improves communication among the physician, patient, and family, and helps with making an accurate diagnosis and planning treatment."[7] Nevertheless, as on any team, there can be harmful members. One of my most important roles as a family physician was helping to empower patients to "fire" family members or friends who negatively affected their health and well-being. In his book *Don't Let Jerks Get the Best of You*, Christian psychiatrist Paul Meier talks in detail about removing the influence of negative family or friends[8]—as does Jan Silvious in her book *Fool-Proofing Your Life.*[9]

Take a Spiritual Inventory

Finding a doctor and other healthcare team members who share your spiritual foundation and practices may be crucial for you—and it's fairly simple. You can use a spiritual inventory to evaluate whether you are on the same page with a member of your team. Here are a few questions you could ask at your interview of a prospective healthcare professional or during your first official appointment. You could come up with some of your own to add.

1. Are you willing to consider my spiritual preferences as you care for me?

2. Are you open to discussing the religious or spiritual implications of my healthcare?

3. Are you willing to work with my spiritual mentors (pastor, priest, rabbi, lay leader) and other members of my

healthcare team (family, friends, mentor, support group) in providing the best possible healthcare?

4. Are you willing to pray with me—or for me—if I feel the need for prayer?

Conclusion

Congratulations! You've done it. By just reading these ten essentials, you've traveled down a road that few people take—a pathway toward applying the essentials of becoming a highly healthy person. This is a great start, but there is even more. We have dozens of evidence-based health and fitness tips to share with you that may well affect the quality and quantity of your life. No person will be able to apply all the principles in this book in a few days or weeks. But you don't have to. We suspect it would take the average person a year or more to apply most of these tips on a consistent basis. So here's your homework.

Set Goals

In your journal, select a page and make two columns. Over the left column write, *Things I've Done or Am Doing.* Over the right column write, *Things I Need to Do.* Then consider what you've accomplished and where you've fallen short. Enter each item in one column or the other. Then look through the left column. What needs improvement and how and when can you improve on these things? Make notes to yourself.

Now look at the right column. Number the items and begin with the item easiest to accomplish and then add more difficult tasks.

Go through the list again and be sure your goals and plans are as specific as possible. The more specific you are about your destination, the more likely you are to arrive. Now choose a date by which you want to accomplish each goal. Be sure to give yourself plenty of time to accomplish each. Accomplishing the goals—even slowly—is much more important than setting goals you can't reach. Write next to the item the date when you expect to accomplish each goal.

Remember, you are a work in progress. Don't obsess. Instead, relax and use your goals and plans to discover and reinforce what is important in your life.

Recruit Assistance and Accountability

Over the next few weeks, review these goals with one or two members of your healthcare team—keeping two things in mind:

- Ask your teammates to review the suitability of your goals, priorities, and timetable. If they don't seem appropriate, adjust them.

- Ask your teammates which goals they'd be willing to help you achieve.

With accountability and assistance, you're more likely to become a highly healthy person.

Have Fun!

You're already on your way to becoming highly healthy. Relax and plan to have fun. Just starting down this road is a tremendous accomplishment. As you look back through your goals and plans, seek those that would be the most fun for you to complete. Go ahead—move them to the top of your list! The more fun you have working toward your health goals, the more likely you are to become highly healthy. Seek ways you can combine goals and plans. For example, if you stop smoking, save the money you spent on cigarettes and treat yourself to a vacation six months later. If you lose weight, treat yourself by purchasing new clothing. The bottom line: enjoy the process. Choosing legitimate plans and goals that are fun can be a great motivator.

Don't Become Discouraged

If you follow these steps, most of your goals will be reachable. Even if you achieve only half of your goals, you'll be well down the road to becoming healthier. Don't become discouraged. If you can't meet a goal, talk it over with one of the members of your healthcare team and then reset your goal. Over time, you can reach them all—one at a time.

PART TWO

22 TIPS FOR A HAPPIER, HEALTHIER YOU

In exercise terms, *reps* or *repetitions* are repeated practices, drills, or training maneuvers designed to make you stronger, faster, more flexible, and healthier. For our tips, we're using the acrostic *REPS* to represent Relational Health, Emotional/Mental Health, Physical Health, and the most important of all, Spiritual Health.

RELATIONAL
HEALTH TIPS

1

TEND TO OTHERS: LOVE YOUR NEIGHBOR

Jesus told a legal expert, "The second [greatest commandment in the Law] is…'Love your neighbor as yourself'" (Matthew 22:39).

Most folks think of neighbors as the people who live near us, but that's not what Jesus meant. Jesus told His famous parable of the good Samaritan to make it clear that "love your neighbor" (Luke 10:25-37) means to love all persons, everywhere—not just our friends and those who live near us.

By "neighbor," Jesus included all mankind—even our enemies! He made this clear when He taught, "You have heard that it was said, 'Love your neighbor and hate your enemy.' But I tell you, love your enemies and pray for those who persecute you, that you may be children of your Father in heaven" (Matthew 5:43-45).

We believe that loving our neighbor encompasses these ideas:

1. forgiving our neighbor

2. following the Golden Rule with our neighbor

3. helping our neighbor in need

We explained the health benefits of forgiveness in essential 3. And we think most folks understand the benefits of the Golden Rule. It may be one of the best-known of Jesus's sayings and sums up His moral teachings, as well as the Law and the Prophets: "So in everything, do to others what you would have them do to you" (Matthew 7:12). This is the standard Jesus set for dealing with our neighbors—in other words, with all people. It is called *The Golden Rule* because Roman Emperor Alexander Severus (AD 222–35) is said to have had it inscribed in gold on his wall.[1]

However, we want to focus on helping our neighbors in need. We are not meant to live hard-hearted or self-centered lives. We are called to put our faith into practice and truly love our neighbors, especially those less fortunate. In what is called *the parable of the sheep and goats*, Jesus taught:

> The King will say to those on His right, "Come, you who are blessed of My Father, inherit the kingdom prepared for you from the foundation of the world. For I was hungry, and you gave Me something to eat; I was thirsty, and you gave Me drink; I was a stranger, and you invited Me in; naked, and you clothed Me; I was sick, and you visited Me; I was in prison, and you came to Me."

> Then the righteous will answer Him, saying, "Lord, when did we see You hungry, and feed You, or thirsty, and give You drink? And when did we see You a stranger, and invite You in, or naked, and clothe You? And when did we see You sick, or in prison, and come to You?"

> And the King will answer and say to them, "Truly I say to you, to the extent that you did it to one of these brothers of Mine, even the least of them, you did it to Me" (Matthew 25:34-45 NASB).

God has given each of us stewardship over what I call *The Four Ts:* our talents (Ephesians 2:10), treasure (Haggai 2:8), time (Ephesians 5:16), and temple—our bodies, the temple of the Holy Spirit (1 Corinthians 6:19). We are to faithfully administer these for our needs and in the service of others. The Bible tells us, "God will generously provide all you need. Then you will always have everything you need and plenty left over to share with others" (2 Corinthians 9:8 NLT).

The unwise say, "The more I give to others, the poorer I become," but the opposite is true. Service to others brings meaning and fulfillment to our lives in a way that wealth, power, possessions, and self-centered pursuits can never match. As Jesus said, "Give, and it will be given to you. A good measure, pressed down, shaken together and running over, will be poured into your lap. For with the measure you use, it will be measured to you" (Luke 6:38).

A biblical principle for a happy (blessed) and healthful life comes with understanding that all God has given us is to be used by us for His glory—and this happens most lavishly when we freely give it back to Him for others' benefit. As with the first disciples, God has given us much to share with those in need. As we do, we can be conduits of healing and blessing every day. We received these blessings freely, and freely we are called to give them away—all for the glory of God. Jesus taught us, "Let your light shine before others, that they may see your good deeds and glorify your Father in heaven" (Matthew 5:16).

John 3:16 tells us that "God so loved the world that He gave…" This verse is a revelation of the heart of God and a summation of the meaning of the Christian life. If there's one thing the Bible teaches us, it's that God is love, and that those of us who claim to believe in Him and want to follow Him ought to love one another as He has loved us (1 John 4:8,11). And the message of John 3:16 is that love always gives—and that God gives sacrificially and maximally.

So what time, talent, and treasure has God given you beyond your basic needs? A devotional from Newspring Church encourages us: "Ask God to tell you how, where, and to whom you can freely give them away. As you use them to serve others, you will experience the blessed life."[2] Randy Alcorn writes, "God has entrusted us with wealth that we may voluntarily distribute to those who need it most. Never have so many been in need. Never has God showered such abundance on Christians. When will we learn that God doesn't give us more to increase our standard of living, but to increase our standard of giving?[3]

From improving your physical well-being to boosting your emotional and relational health, tending to, caring for, and giving to others (loving others) does a world of good for your health and the health of those in which you invest time, treasure, talent, and temple. Most of the time, you can experience the immediate impact of giving your talents, treasure, and time; but it won't be until heaven that we'll learn of all the eternal benefits.

2

VOLUNTEER–FOR YOUR HEALTH

We can share our Four Ts with others in two ways. One is in our vocational work. We can be paid to share our Four Ts. But perhaps the healthiest and most Christlike way is to give away our Four Ts by volunteering. Keep in mind what Paul wrote: "In everything I did, I showed you that by this kind of hard work we must help the weak, remembering the words the Lord Jesus himself said: 'It is more blessed to give than to receive'" (Acts 20:35).

Science backs up the teaching of Jesus. For example, one study found that 75 percent of those who volunteered said volunteering made them feel emotionally happier and physically healthier.[1] A much larger study involving more than 64,000 folks age 60 and older suggested volunteering slows the cognitive decline of aging. An individual who is volunteering 100 hours a year scores on average about 6 percent higher in cognitive testing than a nonvolunteer.[2]

Volunteering makes an immeasurable difference in the lives of others. But it also benefits the volunteer—from lowering stress to boosting self-confidence—especially for older adults. Here are just a few of the mental and physical health benefits of volunteering according to AARP's volunteer program, Create the Good,[3] and the online educational community, Non-Profit Hub:[4]

1. *Reduces stress levels and decreases your risk of depression.*
   Volunteering increases social interaction and helps build

a support system—both of which have been shown to decrease depression. Also, by serving others, volunteers feel a sense of meaning and appreciation—both given and received—which can be calming and reduce depression.

2. *Helps you stay physically and mentally active.* A study released by Johns Hopkins University in 2009 revealed that volunteers increased their brain functioning.[5] Volunteer activities get folks moving and thinking at the same time.

3. *Provides an opportunity to experience the "happiness effect."* Researchers at Vanderbilt University found "the more hours of volunteer work, the greater a person's happiness, life satisfaction, self-esteem, sense of mastery, and physical health, and the lower his or her depression."[6]

4. *Expands connections and boosts self-esteem.* Volunteering helps build a strong safety net for when the volunteer experiences trying times. With strong social ties, the volunteer is surrounded by a community that's willing to help them out when times get tough. Larger social networks provide more resources, which leads to better physical, mental, and emotional health. When you volunteer, you become a part of someone else's safety net too. By helping others, you'll build a greater sense of trust and self-esteem.

5. *Contributes to a longer life.* Volunteers experience increased longevity and less heart disease—and may be at a lower risk for memory loss. Social interaction can significantly reduce the progress of Alzheimer's and other types of dementia.

6. *Gives purpose.* As people get older, they experience a higher risk for isolation. Volunteering combats that by adding a sense of purpose.

7. *Provides a good example.* Volunteering as a family is a

great way to teach important lessons to your children and grandchildren.

Dr. J. Nick Pitts writes, "Elizabeth Andrew put it well when she said volunteers don't necessarily have the time, but they do have the heart. Volunteers give, but in turn end up getting far more. Our time volunteering in schools blessed me more than my organizational skills helped them. My time volunteering in hospitals shaped me more than my mediocre delivery skills assisted them. In the economy of God, you give sacrificially but you gain immeasurably."[7] And, it improves your physical well-being while boosting your emotional and relational health.

Some of the *most* rewarding things we have done in our own lives have been volunteering to help others. We have worked earthquake, tornado, and hurricane recovery. We have volunteered for mission trips to build facilities, as well as to teach pastors and Christian physicians about teaching and sharing their faith in their practices. We have volunteered by distributing gifts to poor children and to the children of prisoners. We have volunteered to teach, to preach, and to clean up church grounds and other places. You may have done some of these things too. Wasn't it rewarding?

Most of the readers of this book have been given a great deal. We have had opportunities that are the envy of the developing world— opportunities to learn, to travel, to make choices that are not available everywhere. Scripture tells us, "From everyone who has been given much, much will be demanded; and from the one who has been entrusted with much, much more will be asked" (Luke 12:48). We have been given much, and we need to be good stewards of what we have received. When we volunteer, we give our time, energy and talents for the benefit of others—we lay down our own lives.

You probably already have volunteer experience. We have found that some volunteering efforts suit us better than others. Our aim in choosing what we volunteer to do is to match the task to our God-given talents and maximize the impact of our work, knowing that volunteering may not only allow us to help others in the name of Christ, but will surely help us be healthier!

3

GET A WORKOUT BUDDY OR BUDDIES

More than 30 years ago, Phil's wife, Brenda, was a young mother with a little daughter, and her friends were young mothers with small children too. These circumstances can make getting in a regular workout a real challenge! Brenda partnered with her friend, Sandy, to run about three miles three days per week. They did it early in the morning, rain or shine.

You see, Brenda didn't want to let Sandy down, and Sandy didn't want to let Brenda down. The positive social pressure compelled them to be regular in getting their exercise. Of all the ways to become more consistent in exercise, getting a workout partner may be the most effective for the most people.

Finding a Workout Buddy

The biggest challenge is to find a good workout partner. Phil has been running regularly for more than 40 years, and most of those runs have been with a workout buddy. He spent his first three years running with a Navy friend who was a fellow competitor in marathons. He was transferred to Virginia, where he ran with another competitor. From there he moved to graduate school to study exercise science, where he found lots of running buddies. After graduation, he joined the faculty at the University of Alabama, where he ran with colleagues and many of his graduate students. Many of his closest friends came from among those workout buddies.

Do you see a pattern here? Most likely your best workout partners will be drawn from people who have the same goals you do—competitive or not—and who are conveniently located. Obviously, your workout schedules must match up. At each stage of Phil's running career, his best workout buddies had similar goals, whether competitive or fitness, and similar schedules.

A practical workout schedule is requisite. As Brenda's example illustrates, early mornings may be the best time to exercise. The earlier in the day we schedule anything, the fewer things can come up to interfere. The next best times, in order, are lunch hour and immediately after work. Experiment and find a time that will work for you and your buddy.

Some types of workouts are more social than others. Running mile after mile lends itself to extended conversations. Swimming mile after mile does not. When weight lifting with free weights, your partner is also your spotter. Being somewhat similar in strength means less changing of weights, which will speed the workout. One caveat we recommend is that you *only* consider a workout partner of the same sex unless they are your spouse.

Experiment

Remember, you are "a design of one by One"! You may be one of those people who prefers to work out alone; and if you can be consistent in exercising alone, good for you. You may find that a workout buddy just doesn't mesh, and that's okay.

However, for most people, working out with others is far more effective. Studies show group workouts provide so much more than just physical benefits. They also support mental and emotional health. Jack Raglin, a professor in the School of Public Health at Indiana University, Bloomington, says "Group exercise or team sports might also have an edge over other forms of exercise because they add an element of accountability." His research has shown that couples who start an exercise program together had a lower dropout rate than those who started one on their own. He adds, "The study showed that very simple forms of social support can be beneficial."[1]

A 2018 study from CDC researchers reported that popular team sports have a slight edge over the other forms of physical activity. The CDC evaluated survey data from 1.2 million adults and reported that "people who exercised reported fewer days of bad mental health than those who didn't. And those who played team sports reported the fewest."[2]

So even if you're someone who usually works out by yourself, perhaps it's time to consider that you may benefit even more from working out in a class or with a buddy or two.

Wise King Solomon taught, "Two are better than one, because they have a good return for their labor: if either of them falls down, one can help the other up. But pity anyone who falls and has no one to help them up" (Ecclesiastes 4:9-10).

The goal is to figure out the best way to do a good workout and do it consistently.

4

REDISCOVER
SEX–WITH
YOUR SPOUSE

A study in the *British Medical Journal* reports that, overall, men with the most active sex lives have a death rate half that of those with the least active (at least during the time period of the study). "There's almost nothing better for you than regular sex. Judging from the many studies on the subject, a daily romp is healthier than yoga, a five-mile run, and a handful of multivitamins combined," writes columnist Tucker Carlson. "Sex has been shown to ameliorate (problems with) memory, posture, depression, anxiety, insomnia, menstrual cramps, digestion, bladder control, dental health, and the sense of smell. It's a natural analgesic that also reduces the risk of prostate cancer and heart disease. It lessens the incidence of colds and flu. It burns calories. Sex prolongs life."[1]

A healthy sex life is even better for devout believers. A comprehensive study of American sexual behavior (*The Social Organization of Sexuality*, published by the University of Chicago in 1994) found "having a religious affiliation was associated with higher rates of orgasm for women...The devout are actually having better sex."[2]

According to the University of Chicago National Health and Social Life Survey, "one of the most comprehensive and methodically sound sex studies ever done," researchers "found that consistent church attendees have a significantly higher frequency and intensity of orgasms than the general population of the US." They also found "church goers not only experience more personal satisfaction but also rate their sex partners as 'extremely enjoyable' significantly more often than other demographics."[3]

Patrick Fagan, a senior fellow at the Family Research Council, said, "Those (married couples) who worship God weekly have the best sex."[4] In other words, monogamous sex in marriage is a pathway to a happier, healthier life.

"As you age, sex isn't the same as it was in your 20s—but it can still be satisfying," write Mayo Clinic experts. "Contrary to common myths, sex isn't just for the young. Many seniors continue to enjoy their sexuality into their 80s and beyond." They add, "A healthy sex life not only is fulfilling, but also is good for other aspects of your life, including your physical health and self-esteem [emotional health]."[5]

Unfortunately, as we age, health issues can impact our sex lives and sexual performance. Chronic health conditions, such as heart disease or arthritis, make sex and intimacy more challenging. Certain surgeries and many medications, such as blood pressure medications, antihistamines, antidepressants, and acid-blocking drugs, can affect sexual function. As a woman ages, her estrogen levels drop, her pelvic organs change, and her natural lubrication for sexual intercourse decreases. For a man, testosterone levels decline, erectile dysfunction increases, and changes in sexual function are common, including:

- a need for more stimulation to achieve and maintain erection and orgasm;
- shorter orgasms;
- less forceful ejaculation and less semen ejaculated; and
- longer time needed to achieve another erection after ejaculation.

But don't give up. You and your partner can experiment with ways to adapt to these natural changes, and your PCP can give you suggestions. Special lubricants for her, erectile dysfunction medications or techniques for him, HT for one or both, and different positions and times for sex for you both can be discussed with your doctor.

A remarkable book, *The Normal Bar: The Surprising Secrets of Happy Couples and What They Reveal About Creating a New Normal in Your Relationship*,[6] describes the results of an online study of 70,000 people from 24 countries. The authors compared couples who said that they had a great sex life compared to couples who said they had a bad sex life. Relationship specialist psychologist John Gottman took their results and his own research studies on more than 3,000 couples over four decades and combined this into a list of 13 things all couples in all countries who have an amazing sex life do:[7]

1. They say "I love you" every day and mean it.

2. They kiss one another passionately for no reason.

3. They give surprise romantic gifts.

4. They know what turns their partners on and off erotically.

5. They are physically affectionate, even in public.

6. They keep playing and having fun together.

7. They cuddle.

8. They make sex a priority, not the last item of a long to-do list.

9. They stay good friends.

10. They can talk comfortably about their sex life.

11. They have weekly dates.

12. They take romantic vacations.

13. They are mindful about "turning toward." Dr. Gottman writes, "In short, they turn toward one another with love and affection to connect emotionally and physically. In the Normal Bar study, only 6% of non-cuddlers had a good sex life…What is very clear from the Normal Bar study is that having a great sex life is not rocket science. It is not difficult."[8]

Finally, Mayo Clinic has these senior sex tips:[9]

- *Talk with your spouse.* Even if it's difficult to talk about sex, openly sharing your needs, desires, and concerns can help you both enjoy sex and intimacy more.

- *Expand your definition of sex.* Intercourse is only one way to have a fulfilling sex life. Touching, kissing, and other intimate contact can be rewarding for you both. Be open to finding new ways to enjoy sexual contact and intimacy.

- *Adapt your routine.* Simple changes can improve your sex life. Change the time of day you have sex to a time when you have the most energy. Try the morning—when you're refreshed from a good night's sleep—rather than at the end of the day.

- *The importance of romance.* Don't give up on it. Because it might take longer for you or your spouse to become aroused, take more time to set the stage for romance. Try a new sexual position or explore other ways of connecting romantically and sexually.

And don't give up on holding hands and hugging. Some studies indicate hugging helps us feel connected and keeps us from getting sick;[10] can reduce stress, slow down the heart and lower blood pressure;[11] and can alleviate fear and anxiety.[12] Hugs can increase healing; increase oxytocin and serotonin levels; relax muscles; while making us feel safe, serene, and happy.[13] Researchers at Carnegie Mellon University found "a hug from a friend or loved one really does help improve your mood if you're having a bad day." They add, "People who consider themselves 'huggers' also have better overall health and stronger relationships."[14]

Prominent family therapist Virginia Satir notes: "We need four hugs a day for survival. We need eight hugs a day for maintenance. We need twelve hugs a day for growth."[15]

"Great sex is not rocket science," says Dr. Gottman. "By being good friends, by being affectionate (yes, even cuddling), and by talking openly about sex, couples can build a thriving relationship inside and outside of the bedroom."[16]

To that end, the Gottman Institute (founded by Drs. John and Julie Gottman) has a resource you might want to check out: a mobile app consisting of more than 100 questions to ask a wife and another 100 questions to ask a husband about each person's "brake and accelerator" when it comes to intimacy (tinyurl.com/ybxu6sam).

My wife, Barb, and I also like and frequently recommend the book *Intimacy Ignited: Discover the Fun and Freedom of God-Centered Sex* by Joseph and Linda Dillow and Peter and Lorraine Pintus,[17] which is a wonderful verse-by-verse look at the Song of Songs and can suggest ways to fire up and maintain the flames of a passionate marriage.

We also recommend *Passion Pursuit: What Kind of Love Are You Making?*[18] by Linda Dillow and Dr. Juli Slattery, which lets God's Word speak about sex as being holy and erotic, blessed by God, and satisfying far beyond what the world can even imagine.

EMOTIONAL
HEALTH TIPS

5

GET A PET—OR TWO!

About two-thirds of US households own at least one pet.[1] About 44 percent of all households in the US have a dog and 35 percent have a cat.[2] Millions of pet owners in the US attest to the joy and companionship their animals provide and know how much their animal friend improves their quality of life. But did you know there are lots of other benefits of pet ownership? The CDC reports that the bond between people and their pets can:[3]

- increase fitness due to increased exercise;
- lower stress, perhaps in part due to increased outdoor activities;
- decrease blood pressure, cholesterol levels, triglyceride levels; and
- decrease feelings of loneliness and increase opportunities for socialization.

Research shows owning a dog may prolong your life and reduce your risk of dying from cardiovascular disease,[4] boost your immune system,[5] improve your fitness, reduce obesity,[6] and reduce stress.[7] In older folks, dog ownership is associated with reduced social isolation and improved perception of well-being.[8] Dog parks are becoming more prevalent, so taking your dog to the park offers opportunities for socialization, which is vital for folks over 50!

One study followed more than 2,500 older adults for three years and found those who regularly walked their dogs "walked faster and for longer time periods each week than others who didn't walk regularly" and "older dog walkers also had greater mobility inside their homes than others in the study."[9] Another study of adults who had suffered a heart attack, reported that a year later, "dog owners were significantly more likely to still be alive than were those who did not own dogs, regardless of the severity of the heart attack."[10]

There has been less research on cat owners, but one study concluded cat owners had a decreased risk for death due to cardiovascular disease (e.g., heart attack and stroke). The researchers suggested acquiring a cat "may represent a novel strategy for reducing the risk of cardiovascular diseases in high-risk individuals."[11] In another study cats "contribute to better psychological health."[12]

If you don't have a pet, should you get a dog or a cat? One study comparing cat and dog owners reported, "The main finding was that owning a dog demonstrated several health-related characteristics to a higher positive degree than both non-pet and cat ownership…Cat owners showed higher body mass index (BMI) values and higher systolic blood pressure and reported worse general health status. They also exercised to a lower degree." The study authors admitted that the results may have been due "to unrelated confounding factors."[13] However, another study of people 50 or older also found that cat owners had a higher BMI, less activity, and shorter duration of activity than dog owners.[14]

There can also be a downside to pets. The *Harvard Health Letter* warns:[15]

> It's not always easy caring for pets, however, and sometimes having them in the home poses health hazards for older adults. If you have problems with gait and stability and your pet can get under your feet or jump up and knock you over, then falls and broken bones are a real danger. There are also sanitary risks associated with pet ownership. Animals can carry parasites that can be transferred to humans…Animal feces carry all kinds of bacteria that can

make you sick. Dogs and cats can also cause allergic reactions in some pet owners.

It's important to note that the likelihood of catching a disease from your pet is low, particularly if precautions are taken. Nevertheless, what can you do to prevent pet-related infections? *Medical News Today* advises:[16]

- *Wash your hands.* Hygiene is key for preventing pet-related infections. After coming into contact with pets, their saliva, or feces, wash hands thoroughly with warm soapy water.

- *Pick up and dispose of feces.* Quickly disposing of your pet's feces, particularly in areas where children play—can prevent the spread of disease to humans and other animals. Wash your hands after doing so.

- *Avoid scratches and bites.* Minimize the risk of infections from pet bites and scratches by avoiding them in the first place. But, if you are scratched, clean the wound immediately with warm soapy water.

- *Get your pet vaccinated and evaluated.* Visit a veterinarian regularly to ensure your pet is healthy and up to date with required vaccinations.

Harvard also advises:[17]

> Before getting a pet, consider if you're physically and mentally able to care for it. Do you have the energy, strength, and mobility to feed it, play with it, clean up after it, and, in the case of dogs, take it for twice-daily walks? Do you have the financial means to pay for pet food and visits to the veterinarian?…The average pet owner spends about $500 to $1,600 per year.

> If you feel you have the physical, mental, and financial means to care for a pet, take the pet's size into consideration—not too big and not too small. Avoid puppies,

which require a great deal of training, time, and energy—
just like having a new baby. And consider the animal's per-
sonality. You don't want a dog that will bark all night or
have a lot of separation anxiety if you leave the house.

Consider finding a rescue pet to adopt. The Society for the Prevention of Cruelty to Animals (SPCA) does not recommend buying or res-
cuing a cat or dog from a pet store. You can read their reasons at tinyurl
.com/y7davta7. However, Best Friends points out, "As awareness of the
connection between puppy mills and puppies sold for profit continues to grow, pet stores across the country are changing the way they do
business. Instead of selling puppies who come from inhumane puppy
mills, and supporting their cruel breeding practices, many stores are
now partnering with local shelters and rescue groups to offer homeless
pets for adoption."[18] They provide a list of humane pet stores in each
state at tinyurl.com/y7vdbzm5.

As kids, most of us had pets for many reasons, but what we didn't
realize were that these pets likely enhanced our health! They still can.
So, if you don't currently have a pet, give it thought—it just might help
your health too.

6

GET OUTDOORS

If you are over 50 and grew up anywhere other than a large city, you likely spent a lot of your early years roaming through neighborhoods, parks, forests, and mountains. We and our siblings grew up in the outdoors, and that may explain our love for it. But it turns out, being outdoors is also highly healthy.

Japanese researchers are describing *shinrin-yoku*, which means taking in the forest atmosphere or "forest bathing," as "the practice of spending time in a forested area in an effort to reap wellness rewards."[1] One study found that participants who walked in a forest had lower blood pressure, reduced pulse, and 15 percent lower stress hormone concentrations than those who strolled through a city environment.[2] Business Insider reports, "Other studies have shown that walking in the woods can improve blood pressure, boost mental health, and decrease cancer risk."[3]

Research published in the *Journal of Positive Psychology* in 2019 found that "participants who sat in an urban park for just five minutes showed significant increases in positive emotions compared to participants who sat in a windowless laboratory room." Of interest, a "second study of 70 students found that spending 15 minutes in nature—rather than just five—did not magnify the effect." Study coauthor, Katherine D. Arbuthnott, said, "When you need an emotional boost, the fastest and easiest way is to spend a few minutes with nature. Actually, being outside is the best, but even contemplating a picture of a natural scene will make a difference."[4]

Other scientists have found that being in nature or going on nature walks has memory-, vision-, and focus-promoting effects while reducing stress, inflammation, fatigue, depression, and anxiety.[5] Nature walks have memory-promoting effects and also boost levels of happiness.[6] Being in nature reduces stress, fatigue, and anxiousness.[7] Another study suggested that relative to energy, spending 20 minutes outside was equivalent to one cup of coffee.[8] A research review reported studies pointing out that natural sunlight helps mitigate pain, and that being outdoors may boost your immune system, may enhance creativity, and "helps us shrug off societal pressures, allowing us to remember and value more important things like relationships, sharing, and community" while "providing free aromatherapy."[9]

Research from the *Journal of the American Heart Association* in 2018 suggested individuals "who live in neighborhoods with more green spaces may have less stress, healthier blood vessels, and a lower risk of heart attacks and strokes than residents of communities without many outdoor recreation areas." The investigators found that "compared to people in areas with the least amount of green space, residents of the greenest neighborhoods had lower urinary levels of the hormone epinephrine, indicating lower stress levels."[10]

Even in city environments, clean, green public spaces make people happier. Researchers "found reductions in feelings of worthlessness, hopelessness and overall poor mental health" when people spent time in vacant lots that had either been "cleaned up" or "greened up."[11]

Despite the benefits of being outdoors, the National Human Activity Pattern Survey reported "Americans spend 87% of their time indoors and an additional 6% in an enclosed vehicle (on average)."[12] In other words, only 7 percent of their day was outside. Yet, one review of ten studies found "getting outside—and moving—for as little as five minutes at a time improved both mood and self-esteem. Exercise near a body of water had the biggest effect."[13] A Stanford study found that "creative thinking improves while a person is walking and shortly thereafter."[14] For this reason, Aristotle created the *peripatetic school,* where students could walk with teachers as they discussed matters.

A study focused on more than 3,000 people at ages 70, 78, 85, and

90 found that those who left the house frequently (six or seven days a week) had a higher chance of living "to the next age group." The results remained the same when researchers accounted for "medical or mobility issues." Dr. Jeremy Jacobs of Hadassah-Hebrew University Medical Center, the study's lead author, said, "There's something about interacting with the world outside that helps."[15]

According to Evan Fleischer, a contributing writer for Big Think, "Doctors in Shetland, Scotland, have been authorized to prescribe nature to their patients. It's thought to be the first program of its kind and seeks to reduce blood pressure and anxiety and increase happiness for those with diabetes, a mental illness, stress, heart disease, and more."[16] The Scottish also believe spending time in nature reduces aggression, attention-deficit/hyperactivity disorder symptoms, improves pain control and the immune system. Fleischer adds, "There's much more we don't know and are figuring out every day."[17]

For followers of Jesus, these data should be no surprise. Dr. J. Nick Pitts has wisely pointed out, "As those who have eyes to see, nature reminds us that we have a purpose in this life, a Provider during this life, and a Sustainer throughout this life (Psalm 8:1-9; Matthew 6:25-34; Colossians 1:15-17). Nature makes us happier because the very rocks will cry out about the one who died to make us more than happy (Luke 19:40)."[18] He adds, "Jesus often used the world as his classroom, taking objects and events and turning them into object lessons. From fig trees to flowers in the field, his renewed mind found the fingerprints of his father everywhere (Mark 11:12-25)."[19]

As Paul observed, "[God's] invisible attributes, namely, his eternal power and divine nature, have been clearly perceived, ever since the creation of the world, in the things that have been made. So they are without excuse" (Romans 1:20 ESV). Nature is, along with Scripture, a tutor, teaching us about the God who created us and everything in the world.

We are primarily outdoor exercisers. Phil runs outside because he likes it so much more than anything he can do inside. Barb and I walk and hike outdoors almost daily. We love it. But you may be different. You may prefer the treadmill, stationary cycle, or rowing machines.

Your schedule or living situation may require indoor exercise. But we encourage you to get outside whenever you can.

What we like about getting outdoors is the variety. Every day is different. There are myriad walking, running, or cycling routes to select. In most of the US, the seasons bring a different perspective on even the same routes. You can change the elevation on a treadmill for variety, but if you live in any part of the country with hills, you are going to get the elevation change just by moving outside.

Being outside affords us the opportunity to see beautiful trees, flowers, birds, animals, and sunsets. We may see the snow softly hitting the evergreen boughs and feel the snowflakes hitting our faces. We will experience rain, cold, and heat. And those experiences are all good. But the best thing to experience when we are physically active outdoors is God Himself. God made a world full of beautiful trees, bushes, flowers, rocks, clouds, and stars. So even if you prefer to get your exercise indoors, take an opportunity to get outside. Look around. See what God hath done!

7

GET YOUR
MIND IN SHAPE

Have you heard this old joke? There are three signs of old age. The first is loss of memory…and I can't remember the other two.

Ah, age-related memory loss can happen. WebMD contributor Susan Kuchinskas says, "These annoying senior moments are the result of a decline in brain activity that shows up in our 50s and affects almost everyone older than 65."[1] Healthcare professionals still find this adage helpful: "It's normal to forget where you put the car keys; it's not normal to forget what the car keys are for." But what can you do to prevent or delay age-related memory loss or dementia?

When it comes to muscles, the saying "use it or lose it" is accurate. But that saying applies to more than just muscle. If we don't exercise our brains, they will also slowly disappear! And, like muscle, we build our brains by giving them a hearty workout.

According to Harvard Health, studies have shown that you can prevent cognitive decline and reduce the risk of dementia with good health habits:[2]

- *Staying physically active.* Exercise delivers more oxygen to the brain and is associated with improved memory, reasoning abilities, and reaction times. Research has shown people think and learn better when walking or doing other forms of exercise.[3] The American Academy of Neurology looked through hundreds of research studies and released guidelines in 2017 that say exercising at least twice a week may help preserve memory and thinking skills.[4] One study found people who reported light to no exercise experienced a decline equal to ten more years of aging as compared to people who reported moderate to intense exercise.[5]

- *Getting enough sleep.* There is a strong relationship between disturbed sleep and an increased risk for cognitive impairment in older adults.[6]

- *Not smoking.* Smoking is linked to a higher risk of cognitive impairment and dementia in older adults.[7]

- *Having good social connections.* Socializing is good for your brain. People who connect with others generally perform better on tests of memory and other cognitive skills. And, in the long run, people with active social lives are less likely to develop dementia than those more socially isolated.[8]

- *Limiting alcohol.* Researchers reviewing studies published from 1971 to 2011 related to alcohol and cognition in the elderly reported that "low to moderate alcohol intake may protect against cognitive decline and dementia and provide cardiovascular benefits."[9] A Wake Forest study of 3,069 community-living older adults found that "among cognitively normal older adults, moderate alcohol intake (1-2 drinks/day) is associated with 40 percent lower risk of dementia over six years.[10] A British study of more than 9,000 people reported "Abstinence [from alcohol] in midlife was associated with a 45% higher risk of dementia compared with people who consumed between one and 14 units of alcohol per week."[11] Although most research suggests a daily drink of alcohol—a small glass (four to five ounces) of red wine, particularly—could be of benefit to brain health, most studies have found that too much alcohol decreases brain health and increases dementia risk.[12]

- *Eating a balanced diet.* The AARP's Global Council on Brain Health has concluded that a diet rich in fruits and vegetables is associated with better brain health and that eating fish and other seafood seems to improve cognitive function.[13] For example, a 2017 study of nearly 1,000 folks age 55 to 99 reported those eating "at least one serving of leafy greens a day had a slower rate of decline on tests of memory and thinking skills than did people who rarely or never ate these vegetables." They concluded, "Regular consumers of such veggies as kale, spinach, collard greens and lettuce enjoyed a mental edge that was the equivalent of 11 years in age."[14] In addition, the AARP has found excessive amounts of alcohol, saturated fats, and salt are harmful to brain health.[15]

We know that God is extremely concerned about the health of your mind. You are to "love the Lord your God with all your heart and with all your soul and with all your mind and with all your strength" (Mark 12:30), "guard your hearts and minds through Christ Jesus" (Philippians 4:7), and "be transformed by the renewing of your mind. Then you will be able to test and approve what God's will is—his good, pleasing and perfect will" (Romans 12:2). You are to "set your mind on things above, not on earthly things" (Colossians 3:2), and "the mind governed by the Spirit is life and peace" (Romans 8:6). The Hebrew word for heart (*leb*) is used more than 800 times in the Old Testament, but in two-thirds of those uses it's best translated "mind" or "will." Clearly, our minds are designed to be healthy physically, emotionally, and spiritually.

Certain health conditions, if not controlled—such as diabetes, high blood pressure, sleep apnea, depression, and hypothyroidism—can impair cognitive skills. If you have any of these health issues, you can help protect your memory by following your doctor's advice.

Working Out Our Minds

Not only should we exercise our hearts and our muscles, but we also need to exercise our brains. Merely keeping our minds engaged is the most basic step. Reading is an excellent way to keep our brains active, as well as allowing us to learn lots of useful information. And remember that reading Scripture has multiple benefits.

Problem solving is another good brain exercise. The problems can be real ones, such as "How do I encourage my friends to get healthier?" or invented problems, such as crossword puzzles, sudoku, or chess. Another brain-stretcher is Scripture. Deeply understanding Scripture can be a challenge. Phil was part of a group of professors at the US Military Academy who met weekly to discuss the parables of Jesus. This group of educators might have gotten a bit carried away with overanalysis, but they found as many questions as they did answers!

Sandra Bond Chapman, PhD, recommends that adults 55 and older use several simple strategies to regain lost cognitive performance, improve blood flow in the brain, speed up communication between its regions, and expand its structural connections. She says, "Some of these positive changes can be evoked in a matter of hours."[16] Consider these:

1. *Don't try to do too much.* Mental work is good for us, but when we try to accomplish too much at once, we are more prone to make errors and feel stressed. The solution is to make sure we allot time for brain breaks and prioritize our to-do list each day. Place the two most important items, the ones that require the greatest brainpower, at the top of the list. Set aside focused time, away from phone calls, texts, and e-mails, to give undivided attention to the task at hand. Completing our most challenging to-dos delivers a daily sense of accomplishment and allows us to achieve noticeable progress.

2. *Zoom out.* When you are bogged down in details and minutiae, your brain often gets stuck blindly following directions and regurgitating facts. The solution is to take time to step back and get the 10,000-foot view. Achieving a new perspective will inspire your brain to generate new ideas and solutions.

3. *Embrace the unknown.* Curiosity is a powerful force. It
encourages us to continually ask, "What if?" Foster it
by committing to exploring your God-given passions.
Stepping into the unknown does not mean abandoning
what you know and love. Chapman says, "Simply
challenging yourself to broaden and deepen your
knowledge or skill will ensure you and your brain are
constantly changing, growing, and expanding."[17]

According to research published in the journal *Neurology*, "Those
who engaged in mentally stimulating activities...experienced slower
memory decline compared to those who didn't. People who exercised their minds later in life had a 32-percent lower rate of mental
decline compared to their peers with average mental activity. The rate
of decline amongst those with infrequent mental activity, on the other
hand, was 48 percent faster than the average group."[18]

Experts at Harvard tell us, "Challenging your brain with mental
exercise is believed to activate processes that help maintain individual
brain cells and stimulate communication among them. Many people
have jobs that keep them mentally active, but pursuing a hobby, learning a new skill, or volunteering for a project at work that involves a
skill you don't usually use can function the same way and help improve
memory."[19]

"Think of it this way," write Kitty Crenshaw and clinical psychologist Cathy Snapp, PhD, "The act of replacing negative thoughts with
good thoughts physically impacts the synapses in our brain, causing
them to disconnect and make brand-new connections, creating new
pathways and cells devoted to right thinking." They add, "We turbo-
charge the process by engaging in positive lifestyle choices such as exercising and adding nutrient-rich foods to grow healthy brain structure.
Literally, in a process described as *neuroplasticity*, a new brain can be
created to replace the old brain![20] Like Paul wrote, "Be transformed by
the renewing of your mind" (Romans 12:2).

Last, but not least, if you're concerned about your memory, be sure
to see your healthcare professional.

8

ENJOY THE
REWARDS OF AGING

One of the surprises for us about getting older is that we do *not* envy young folks! We both enjoyed our younger days, and in those days had a certain pity for people over 50, but no longer. In fact, our sympathies are directed toward college students who haven't even started building careers or families.

True enough, as we age, our physical abilities will diminish for most of us. We have written this book to minimize the decline and even help some folks improve beyond their younger capacities. The Book of Wisdom tells us, "The glory of the young is their strength; the gray hair of experience is the splendor of the old" (Proverbs 20:29 NLT). So we don't mourn getting a little older.

Psalm 92:12-15 tells us, "The righteous will flourish like a palm tree, they will grow like a cedar of Lebanon; planted in the house of the LORD, they will flourish in the courts of our God. They will still bear fruit in old age, they will stay fresh and green, proclaiming, 'The LORD is upright; He is my Rock, and there is no wickedness in Him.'" These verses carry a commission for us. If we choose righteousness, we will flourish (be highly healthy) and will still bear fruit, staying fresh and green. The tips we have given you are aimed at helping you achieve just that.

An article in *American Family Physician* reported a Gallup poll that "revealed some positive aspects of aging, including overall perception of well-being, fewer worries (less than those in their 20s), and more supportive relationships. The respondents also reported better coping skills, 'positivity bias' in relationships, and improved ability to regulate emotions. Aging, while putting a damper on our physical function and threatening vision and mobility, may still allow for improved well-being, happiness, supportive relationships, humor, and even inspiration for creative writing and poetry."[1]

What about the health effects of retirement? The Bible speaks very little concerning retirement (Numbers 8:23-26), but it does speak of moving into different seasons (Ecclesiastes 3:1-7). You may not need a reason to retire early, but a good one to consider is that it could lengthen your life. One Dutch study showed early retirement by civil servants over the age 54 decreased the probability of death over the following five years by 42 percent compared to those who continued working.[2] An analysis in the US "found about seven years of retirement can be as good for health as reducing the chance of getting a serious disease (like diabetes or heart conditions) by 20 percent."[3] The researchers hypothesized two reasons for this: Retirees have more time to invest in their health, and retirement can reduce stress, which may be why retirees in the study were less likely to die from cardiovascular diseases.[4]

Other research supports later retirement. Researchers in the US and Australia found that, among healthy retirees, "a one-year older age at retirement was associated with an 11 percent lower risk of all-cause mortality." They add, "Early retirement may be a risk factor for mortality, and prolonged working life may provide survival benefits among US adults."[5]

Not all retirees are happy in retirement. A 2016 Employee Benefit Research Institute (EBRI) study analyzed retirement satisfaction trends between 1998 and 2012 and found the percent "very satisfied" dropped from 60 to 49 percent, while those "not at all satisfied" increased from 8 to 11 percent.[6]

New York Times contributor Austin Frakt says, "Research shows a link, but it isn't retirement itself that leads to a longer life. It's what you do in retirement."[7] Retirees are more likely to exercise,[8] get more sleep,[9] and spend more time doing household work and gardening[10]—all of which are more active than a desk job. Another study found that better health in retirement may be because of the reduced likelihood of smoking.[11]

When Phil and Brenda sought counsel on retirement from the university, one statement captured their attention: "Don't retire *from* something, retire *to* something!" And for those seeking retirement, we support that advice. However, if you follow the tips in this book, healthy living doesn't have to start when retirement begins.

Some Options

Throughout this book we have shared things that you can retire *to*, not *from*. We encourage you to continue to travel, to continue to learn and grow. We want you to stay physically and spiritually active. We want you to volunteer. We want you to live wisely and spend your time wisely. And we want you to keep clearly in mind that this world is not our home, and this body is not our final body. Be good stewards of this temple of the Holy Spirit (1 Corinthians 6:19), but never lose sight of the true destination—our heavenly home.

There is no end to the rewards and opportunities of aging. Here are a few:

1. *Tell Stories.* We have stories about a lot of topics. Stories of successes and failures. Our friend, gerontology expert Dr. Mike Parker, encourages people to write their stories. Dr. Parker calls it a "Life Review" and suggests that family members and friends can benefit from a written Life Review.

   One of the easiest ways to do this is found on the website StoryWorth.[12] For a fee, they make it easy and fun for you to share your story with loved ones. They send weekly e-mailed story prompts—including questions you may never have thought about answering—and your stories are e-mailed weekly to any friends or family you want. Then at the end of a year, you'll get the stories bound in a hardcover book.

   Also consider getting a book like *300 Questions to Ask Your Parents Before It's Too Late* and answering those questions yourself for your kids and grands. Strengthen your bond with your family as they get to know you in a whole new way.

2. *Try new things.* Begin your journey of becoming fitter and healthier by identifying the tips of ours, as well as other healthy activities you haven't tried. Try fishing, or knitting, or hiking, or painting. Prioritize them and begin doing one a week or one a month. One of the benefits of aging for many is more discretionary time, so try something new, one tip at a time.

3. *Pray and meditate more.* Ask God to give you opportunities for teaching, service, or missionary work and then listen for His direction…and obey!

4. *Volunteer.* If you've raised children, think back to the work involved. Volunteer to watch someone else's kids, whether it's a neighbor, church member, or one of your own children, and give them a chance to get away for a weekend and strengthen their own marriage. Or, if childcare is not appealing, volunteer in a soup kitchen, in a local Christian service organization, and particularly in your own church congregation. Volunteer to do something new and check two of these items off your to-do list.

PHYSICAL
HEALTH TIPS

9

FIVE HABITS TO LIVE TEN YEARS LONGER (OR MORE)!

The title of this tip sounds incredible, yet it's true. In 2018, the Social Security Administration projected that about 25 percent of today's 65-year-olds will live past 90, with approximately 10 percent living to be older than 95.[1] I've had many a patient who has told me, "Doc, if I'd have known I was going to live this long, I would have taken better care of myself." Well, now you know.

Researchers, using National Health and Nutrition Examination Survey data, reported the life expectancy at age 50 was 29 years for women and 25.5 years for men who *lacked* five specific "low-risk life-style factors." In contrast, those who *had* all five "low-risk factors" projected a life expectancy at age 50 years of about 43 years for women and 38 years for men.[2]

That's a life-expectancy *increase* of 14 years for women and more than 12 years for men, a whopping 48-49 percent increased lifespan for women and men! In addition, three-fourths of premature cardiovascular deaths and half of premature cancer deaths in the US could be attributed to lack of adherence to the five low-risk factors:[3]

1. never smoking
2. a normal weight BMI of 18.5 to 24.9 (see tinyurl.com/qyqhmdx to calculate your BMI)

3. thirty or more minutes per day of moderate-to-vigorous physical activity

4. no or limited alcohol intake

5. a high-quality, nutrient-dense diet

It's clear from scores of studies that the above factors are associated with a lower risk of premature mortality. But, you might argue, the life expectancy of Americans is going up all the time anyway. And that is correct. It has increased from about 63 years in 1940 to about 79 years in 2016.[4] This increase is the result of a number of factors, such as improvements in living standards, improved medical treatment, reduction in smoking, and a modest improvement in diet. But, unfortunately, national surveys show the percent of Americans adhering to a low-risk lifestyle is decreasing. During the last three decades, it has shrunk from 15 percent in the 1990s to 8 percent in the 2000s.[5] A 2018 study by the CDC found that only 23 percent of US adults get enough exercise, whereas a 2017 study reported just one in ten Americans eats sufficient fruits and vegetables.[6]

Therefore, the downward trend in low-risk lifestyles is preventing life expectancy in America from being even higher. Globally, the US ranks forty-third when it comes to life expectancy, according to 2017 data from the Central Intelligence Agency's World Factbook. The three countries ranked highest for life expectancy at birth were Monaco (89.4 years), Japan (85.3 years), and Singapore (85.2 years).[7] The life expectancy in the US is not higher, say researchers at the University of South Carolina, because obesity and moderate alcohol use is increasing, whereas physical activity and consumption of five or more fruits and vegetables a day are decreasing.[8] Obesity in the US is epidemic. A 2019 report by the National Center for Health Statistics showed "that both men and women gained on average a whopping 24 pounds from 1960 to 2002; and, through 2016, men had gained an additional eight pounds, and women another seven pounds."[9]

In addition, although cigarette smoking has gone down (in 2018 cigarette smoking reached the "lowest level ever recorded among US adults"[10]), new forms of smoking have gone up (e-cigarettes or vaping, cigarillos, hookah, clove and menthol cigarettes, etc.). According to the American Cancer Society (ACS), "People often think some forms are safe and don't cause health problems. This isn't true. There is no safe form of tobacco."[11] So smoking is still the leading cause of preventable disease and death in the US, accounting for about one in five deaths.[12]

If you're in the 8 percent of Americans who meet all five low-risk factors, congratulations! If you're not, the tips in this book are for you.

10

YOU NEED TO KNOW FOUR NUMBERS

A study published in 2018 in the *Journal of the American Heart Association* reported the number of people with an ideal cardiovascular health score, based on seven lifestyle and biological measures,* decreased from 8.5 to 5.9 percent over the last 20 years. Researchers said the decrease was due to poorer scores for blood pressure, blood cholesterol, blood sugar (also called blood *glucose*), and BMI.[1]

The CDC reports 40 million Americans are living with uncontrolled high blood pressure,[2] 39 million adults aren't taking the recommended statin therapy to manage their cholesterol,[3] more than 100 million have poor blood sugar control (with diabetes or prediabetes),[4] and more than one-third (over 78 million) are obese, and 71 percent are overweight or obese.[5]

When it comes to these four risk factors, 13 percent of US adults over 35 years old have not had blood pressure screening, 18 percent have not had cholesterol or lipid screening, and 36 percent have not had diabetes or obesity screening.[6]

Although you may know that each of these can increase your risk for disease and premature death—from cardiovascular disease, diabetes, cancer, and other health problems, you may not know how they are linked together and how often you should be evaluated for each.

---

* The American Heart Association created what it calls *Life's Simple 7* in 2010 to help track improvements in the health of Americans. The measures are: tobacco use, diet, physical activity, BMI, blood pressure, total cholesterol, and blood sugar. We have tips on each for you.

The USPSTF, an independent panel of experts in primary care and prevention,[7] and the American Heart Association (AHA), along with other national groups,[8] have a series of recommendations on what we're calling, "You Need to Know Four Numbers."

Blood Pressure

The AHA recommends that all adults 20 or older get their blood pressure checked at least once every two years as long as it is below 120/80 mm mercury (Hg). If either number (the upper number, the systolic blood pressure, or the lower number, the diastolic blood pressure) is higher, check it more often. High blood pressure can be controlled through lifestyle changes and medication.[9] The USPSTF recommends screening for high blood pressure at 18 years of age. Both recommend abnormal tests be confirmed by obtaining blood pressure readings away from the doctor's office—for example, with home blood pressure monitoring—before starting treatment. This is a *key* recommendation because merely being in medical facilities raises some people's blood pressure.[10]

Cholesterol

Cholesterol is a waxy substance your body uses to protect nerves, make cells, and produce certain hormones. Your liver makes all the cholesterol your body needs. Your body also gets cholesterol directly from food (such as eggs, meats, and dairy products). Too much cholesterol negatively impacts your health.

LDL, "bad" cholesterol, delivers cholesterol to the body, whereas HDL removes cholesterol from the bloodstream. This explains why too much LDL cholesterol is bad, and why high HDL cholesterol is good. For example, if your total cholesterol level is high because of a high LDL, you may be at higher risk of heart disease or stroke. But, if your total cholesterol level is high only because of a high HDL, you're probably not at higher risk. So, you want your HDL to be *high* and your LDL to be *low*.

The AHA recommends a lipoprotein profile be taken every four to six years, starting at age 20. This is a blood test that measures total cholesterol, each cholesterol type, and triglycerides. You may need to be tested more frequently if your healthcare provider determines that you're an increased risk for heart disease or stroke. Like high blood pressure, cholesterol can often be controlled through lifestyle changes and medication.[11] The USPSTF recommends lipid testing and calculation of 10-year cardiovascular disease risk in all adults ages 40 to 75 years.[12]

Blood Sugar

High blood sugar (glucose) could mean you have prediabetes or diabetes. Untreated diabetes leads to many serious medical problems including heart disease and stroke. If you're overweight *and* you have at least one additional cardiovascular risk factor, you may need a blood glucose test. There are a couple of options. Your PCP can do a fasting or random blood sugar or a blood test called the *glycated hemoglobin* (or *A1C*) to estimate your risk of prediabetes or diabetes. The great thing about the A1C is that it can tell you your average blood sugar level for the previous three months. The American Diabetes Association recommends regular screening for diabetes starting at age 45, with repeated tests at least every three years.[13] The USPSTF recommends screening for abnormal blood glucose as part of cardiovascular risk assessment in adults aged 40 to 70 years who are overweight or obese.[14]

Weight

You may remember the data from the Harvard School of Public Health on the leading preventable risk factors for premature death in the US. High blood pressure was number two on the list (after smoking), killing about 395,000 Americans each year. Overweight/obesity was number three (killing 216,000), high blood sugar was number five (killing 190,000), and high LDL (bad) cholesterol was number six (killing 113,000). Sedentary behavior (inactivity or inadequate physical activity) was number four (killing 191,000).[15]

The reason we have these together here is because of a common and dangerous disorder called *metabolic syndrome*, which is a set of risk factors for heart disease and premature death—including high blood pressure, high cholesterol, high sugar, and being overweight. What makes it insidious is that metabolic syndrome does not have any true signs or symptoms until it's too late. So how is metabolic syndrome diagnosed?

Your doctor diagnoses metabolic syndrome if at least three of the following are true:[16]

- You are overweight or obese, and you carry the weight around your middle. For men, this means a waist larger than 40 inches and larger than 35 inches for women.
- You have higher-than-normal blood pressure (130/85 mm Hg or higher).
- You have a higher-than-normal blood sugar (a fasting blood sugar of 110 mg/dL or higher).
- You have a higher-than-normal amount of fat in your blood (a triglyceride level of 150 mg/dL or higher).
- You have a lower than normal HDL cholesterol (an HDL less than 40 mg/dL).

The more of these risk factors you have, the higher your risk of heart disease and premature death.

To review, these critical items are the key screening tests for monitoring cardiovascular health:

1. *Blood pressure* every two years as long as the blood pressure is less than 120/80 mm Hg.

2. *Cholesterol as a "fasting lipoprotein profile"* every four to six years for normal-risk people to measure total, HDL, and LDL cholesterol; more often if you have elevated risk for heart disease and stroke.

3. *Blood glucose or A1C test* at least every three years.

4. *Weight/BMI* during each healthcare visit.

5. *Discuss smoking, physical activity, and diet* during each regular healthcare visit.

All our readers should know their numbers: their blood pressure, BMI, cholesterol (that is, lipids, especially LDL), and their FBS (or, better yet, A1C). If you don't have up-to-date numbers, get them ASAP. Your life may depend on it.

11

EAT LIKE A GREEK

What's the best diet overall? What's the best diet for weight loss? What's the best diet for preventing chronic disease—whether cardiovascular disease or inflammatory diseases such as arthritis or diabetes? Everyone has an opinion, but what do the experts say? My favorite answer to these questions comes in the annual ratings from *US News and World Reports*. The editors convene "a panel of food and health experts to rank 40 diets on a variety of measures" such as "the diet's ability to help a person lose weight in the short and long term."[1] What's the best?

Before sharing the best nutrition plans, let us suggest what may be the worst diet in America. (Know that we say this as thoroughly Southern boys!) The most damaging diet, according to a study published in *Journal of the American Medical Association (JAMA)*, is the "Southern-Style Diet"—described as including "fried food, cheesy casseroles, and sweet, sweet tea," as well as "high amounts of salt, sugar, and fat." In fact, the authors describe the diet as "deadly, especially to African-Americans," by increasing "blood pressure up to killer levels."[2] A 2019 study of more than 100,000 postmenopausal women showed "frequent consumption of fried foods, especially fried chicken and fried fish/shellfish, was associated with a higher risk of all cause and cardiovascular mortality in women in the US."[3]

What were the best diets?[4] In 2019 the "Best Diets Overall" and "The Best Diets for Healthy Eating" were the Mediterranean Diet, followed by the DASH Diet and the Flexitarian Diet. In "The Easiest Diet to Follow," the Mediterranean Diet was tops, followed by a second-place tie between the Flexitarian and Weight Watchers diets.

The best three diets for weight loss were, in order: the WW (Weight Watchers) Diet, followed by a second-place tie between the Volumetrics Diet, and the Flexitarian Diet. For the best "Heart-Healthy Diets," the Mediterranean Diet and the Ornish Diet tied for first, followed by the DASH Diet. In the "Best Plant-Based Diet" category, the experts chose, in this order, the Mediterranean Diet, the Flexitarian Diet, with the Nordic and Ornish diets in a third-place tie. In the "Best Commercial Diet Plans," the winners were the WW (Weight Watchers) Diet, the Jenny Craig Diet, and the Nutritarian diet.

We don't think you can go wrong with any of these. In fact, two eating plans—(1) a vegetarian diet that includes eggs and dairy and (2) the Mediterranean diet—were shown to be equally effective in reducing body weight, BMI, and fat mass in a three-month randomized trial of 100 adults. The vegetarian diet was better lowering LDL and the Mediterranean better at lowering triglyceride levels; so, it was concluded, both protected heart health equally.[5]

Our current favorite to recommend is the Mediterranean Diet, followed closely by the Flexitarian and DASH diets, which emphasize consuming lots of fruits and vegetables as well as healthy fatty foods like fish, nuts, and olive oil.[6] According to a CDC report, "The vast majority of Americans are not eating enough fruits and vegetables." That study found only about one in ten American eat the daily recommended amount of fruit, while less than 9 percent ate their daily recommended amount of vegetables.[7]

The American Heart Association says, "Mediterranean-style diets are often close to our dietary recommendations, but they don't follow them exactly. In general, the diets of Mediterranean peoples contain a relatively high percentage of calories from fat. This is thought to contribute to the increasing obesity in these countries, which is becoming a concern."[8]

The 2015–2020 US Dietary Guidelines say, "There are many ways to consume a healthy eating pattern, and the evidence to support multiple approaches has expanded over time. The Healthy

Mediterranean-Style Eating Pattern and Healthy Vegetarian Eating Pattern, which were developed by modifying the Healthy US-Style Eating Pattern, are two examples of healthy eating patterns individuals may choose based on personal preference."[9] You can find more on these at tinyurl.com/yc6nbarz.

The Mediterranean Diet is based upon the general belief that the people in countries bordering the Mediterranean Sea live longer and suffer less chronic disease, cardiovascular disease, and cancer than most Americans. There isn't a specific Mediterranean diet. Italians eat differently from Greeks, who eat differently from the Spanish. But folks in these countries have a not-so-surprising secret: a lifestyle that is active combined with a diet low in red meat, sugar, and saturated fat, while high in produce, nuts, and other healthful foods.[10]

According to the Texas Heart Institute, "Working with the Harvard School of Public Health, Oldways, a nonprofit food think tank in Boston, has developed a consumer-friendly Mediterranean diet pyramid that emphasizes fruits, veggies, whole grains, beans, nuts, legumes, olive oil, and flavorful herbs and spices; eating fish and seafood at least a couple of times a week; enjoying poultry, eggs, cheese, and yogurt in moderation; and saving sweets and red meat for special occasions."[11] According to a 2018 study, "People who followed this type of diet had 25 percent less risk of developing cardiovascular disease over the course of 12 years."[12] You can find additional guidance at tinyurl.com/yazwknqu.

For more information about these healthful diet plans, including their health and nutrition effects, lots of recipes, dos and don'ts, and an expert review on each, here are some websites (in alphabetical order):

1. DASH Diet: tinyurl.com/yd53cmg4

2. Flexitarian Diet: tinyurl.com/ybhdqzly

3. Jenny Craig Diet: tinyurl.com/yckqw3nn

4. Mediterranean Diet: tinyurl.com/ycfrux8b

5. Ornish Diet: tinyurl.com/ydddc8rl

6. Volumetrics Diet: tinyurl.com/y7l6wx8y

7. Weight Watcher's Diet: tinyurl.com/ybqsuf5o

What were the lowest-ranking diets? The panel's bottom ten rankings, from lowest up, were: the Dukan Diet (#41), Body Reset Diet (#40), the Keto Diet tied with the Whole30 Diet (#38), the Atkins Diet (#37), Fast Diet, Paleo Diet, Raw Food Diet, Supercharged Hormone Diet (tied for #33) and the Alkaline Diet (#32).

Combine the healthful diet you choose with staying physically active and the other tips you're learning in this book, and you'll be on your way to better health.

12

MOVE!

I f you're plopped on a bed, couch, or chair right now," write the editors of *Reader's Digest*, "you might have what is arguably the most common health problem in America today—*sitting disease*." That might sound silly. But prolonged sitting—*sedentary living*—has been shown by researchers to play a significant role in many of the most troublesome health issues of our time, from obesity and heart disease to diabetes and depression.[1]

Sitting too much, according to a study from the University of Cambridge, is twice as likely to lead to premature death as being obese![2] Regular exercise increases longevity, reduces fatigue and disability,[3] reduces the risk of heart failure,[4] and improves mental health (with team sports and those involving social groups having the most positive effect on mental health).[5] Being physically fit may reduce the risk of developing glaucoma by nearly 50 percent.[6]

Research, published in the journal *JAMA Network Open*, reported how the Cleveland Clinic studied more than 122,000 patients from 1991 to 2014, putting them under treadmill testing and later recording mortality rates. They reported a clear connection between exercise and a longer, healthier life.[7] "Being unfit on an exercise stress test had a worse prognosis, as far as death, than being hypertensive, being diabetic, or being a current smoker," Cleveland Clinic cardiologist and study author Wael Jaber told CNN. "We've never seen something as pronounced as this and as objective as this."[8] He added that lack of exercise "should be treated as a disease that has a prescription, which is called *exercise*."[9]

Research published in *Circulation* that included almost 500,000 adults ages 40 to 69 linked higher fitness levels to a lower likelihood of heart disease even for people with genetic variants that dramatically increased their cardiovascular risks. The study concluded, "Even if you have a genetic risk for heart disease, there's a simple way to combat it: Exercise!" Among participants determined to have the highest genetic risk for cardiovascular disease, the highest level of cardiorespiratory fitness was associated with a 49 percent lower risk for coronary heart disease![10]

Sitting too much "undermines your metabolic and heart health."[11] Research has associated sedentary behavior to a higher risk of conditions such as heart disease and diabetes, and a greater chance of premature death.[12] Americans are sitting an average of 13 hours a day.[13] Journalist Brigid Schulte of the *Washington Post* cites that some medical researchers have gone so far as to say that "the office chair is worse for your health than smoking and kills more people than HIV."[14]

In that same article, Schulte says, "Experts say you should start standing up at work for at least two hours a day—and work your way toward four," adding, "the average office worker sits for about 10 hours" throughout an average work day.[15] Other researchers found not only that standing burns more calories than sitting, but as senior author Professor Francisco Lopez-Jimenez said, "The additional muscle activity is linked to lower rates of heart attacks, strokes, and diabetes, so the benefits of standing could go beyond weight control."[16]

An 18-year study published in the *European Journal of Preventive Cardiology* found that even low-intensity physical activity such as walking, gardening, and housework can improve your heart health.[17] Psychologist John Hackston writes, "People tend to think that there's one best way to go about an exercise routine, but one-size-fits-all doesn't apply here. Instead, it's important to know who you are and select a type of exercise that fits." He adds, "From a behavior change perspective, the more you enjoy the activity, the more likely you are to stick with it."[18]

Other experts now "believe they have pinpointed the exact amount of time we need to spend working out in order to look after our hearts." Findings published in the *Journal of Physiology* "found varying amounts of exercise can affect different-sized arteries." For instance, "the study found exercising two to three days a week for 30 minutes may help minimize stiffening in middle-sized arteries, while larger central arteries will stay youthful when you exercise four to five days a week."[19]

It should now be very apparent to you that one of the worst things you can do for your health is to do nothing at all. According to *Men's Health Magazine*, with sedentary behavior:[20]

1. *Your mood takes a dive.* Feeling down? It may be your butt! After surveying more than 3,300 government employees, researchers found that men who sat for more than six hours a day at work were 90 percent more likely to feel moderate psychological distress—nervousness, restlessness, hopelessness, or even fatigue—compared to men who sat for less than three hours a day.[21]

2. *Your cancer risk skyrockets.* A German meta-analysis of 43 different studies including more than four million people found that sedentary behavior significantly increases your risk for several types of cancer, including colon, endometrial, and lung cancers.[22]

3. *You start to forget things.* Your brain health suffers when you lounge for too long.[23] Older adults who are sedentary may be just as likely to develop dementia as people who are genetically predisposed to the condition, research published in the *Journal of Alzheimer's Disease* found.[24] A recent study of 11,000 older folks was published in *Neurology* and reported people who exercise about an hour, three days a week, had improved cognition. Walking was the most common exercise. In terms of a possible reason for the observed improvement, a researcher who was not part of the study commented, "Physical activity improves blood circulation all over the body—that includes the brain."[25]

4. *Your blood sugar spikes.* Even if you're at a healthy weight, your blood sugar levels can rise if you're parked in a chair for too long, according to a University of Florida study. In fact, sedentary adults were more likely to have blood sugar levels high enough to be considered prediabetes by the American Diabetes Association.[26]

5. *Your sex life slows down.* Your inactive behavior can lead to your developing a paunch (fat belly) and that might predispose you for sexual problems later. Men with a waist of 42 inches or more are more than twice as likely to have erectile dysfunction (ED) than those with waists below 32 inches, one Harvard study found.[27] After surveying 300 men, researchers in Los Angeles found that highly active men—or men who completed 3.5 hours of moderate exercise or more a week—had higher sexual function scores than men who reported less physical activity.[28]

6. *You'll toss and turn.* Ever feel like you sleep more soundly after logging a great workout? That's because exercising at least 150 minutes a week can improve the quality of your shuteye, according to a study published in *Mental Health and Physical Activity.*[29] In fact, those who exercise are nearly twice as likely to experience a good night's sleep every night compared to people who avoid the gym, a National Sleep Foundation poll found. More than two-thirds of vigorous exercisers reported almost never experiencing symptoms associated with insomnia. In contrast, 50 percent of people who don't exercise reported waking up in the middle of the night.[30]

7. *Your backache gets worse.* Sitting for as little as four hours straight can increase pressure on the disks in your lower back, a Penn State study found.[31] This compression can lead to disk degeneration, a common culprit for back pain. So get up and move, the researchers suggest. When the participants in the study changed their position every

15 minutes, they didn't experience adverse effects in their disks.

Until recently, healthcare professionals felt that the remedy for being sedentary—for what is now called *sitting disease*—was working out, especially with formal exercise sessions. But new research is changing that thinking. As it turns out, just being up and about throughout the day can be as healthy for you as a workout. Twenty minutes of brisk walking each day (even split among more than one walking session) could be enough to reduce an individual's risk of early death, according to a study of more than 334,000 European men and women.[32] Hippocrates said, "Walking is man's best medicine,"[33] and science agrees. *Prevention Magazine* lists these benefits of walking:[34]

1. *Your mood improves.* Regular walking modifies your nervous system so much that you'll experience a decrease in anger and hostility. When you make your walks social— with a friend or your spouse—you feel connected, which boosts mood.

2. *Your creative juices flow.* Research found that the walkers thought more creatively than sitters.

3. *Your jeans get looser.* Regular walking can improve your body's response to insulin, which can reduce belly fat. "Daily walking increases metabolism by burning extra calories *and* by preventing muscle loss, which is particularly important as we get older."[35]

4. *You'll slash your risk of chronic disease.* The American Diabetes Association says walking lowers blood sugar and your risk for diabetes. Researchers found regular walking lowered blood pressure by as much as 11 points and reduced stroke risk by 20 to 40 percent. Another study found those who walked 30 or more minutes on five or more days per week had a 30 percent lower risk of cardiovascular disease, compared with those who did not walk regularly.

5. *Your digestion improves.* A regular walking routine can greatly improve gastric mobility.

6. *When you become a regular walker, you establish a regular routine.* When you have a routine, you are more likely to continue with the activity and take on new healthy behaviors.

Mayo Clinic experts add these benefits about walking:[36]

- Improves your balance and coordination.

- Strengthens your bones and muscles.

We recommend walking because it is simple. Except for certain disabilities and injuries, most of us can walk fine without any coaching. Your 30 minutes of walking doesn't have to be in one session. The CDC says three 10-minute sessions has the same healthful benefits. Park a 10-minute walk from work, walk to and from work, and then walk for 10 minutes before lunch.[37] Bam! You've done your 30 minutes. And 2019 guidelines from the Department of Health and Human Services urges Americans "to exercise even if it is just for a few minutes at a time."[38] According to the updated physical activity guidelines published in *JAMA,* "Even two minutes of any physical activity—taking the stairs, walking the dog, or carrying out the trash—can add up to significant health benefits, such as improved blood pressure, enhanced brain function, and reduced risk of cancer and weight gain."[39]

Another 2019 report concluded, "Sedentary individuals who climbed three flights of stairs three times daily for six weeks, with up to four hours between sessions, showed higher cardiorespiratory fitness, performed better in a maximal cycling test, and were stronger after the intervention, compared with those who did not exercise… They underscore the idea that 'exercise snacks' can improve health."[40] Maybe exercise snacking will be of help to the 77 percent of American adults who are not getting either 150 minutes of moderate exercise or 75 minutes of vigorous exercise each week.[41] The report concluded, "In all, the results suggest that most Americans should try to squeeze more exercise into their time off, given its well-established connections to everything from chronic disease prevention to mental and cognitive health benefits."[42]

A 2015 study found that people who replaced "some of their sitting time with a light-intensity activity like strolling gained a substantial benefit in terms of mortality risk." In fact, if participants "replaced as little as two minutes of sitting each hour with gentle walking, they lowered their risk of premature death by about 33 percent, compared with people who sat almost nonstop."[43] A study in *Circulation* of adults age 45 to 64 suggested that individuals "can make up for years of sedentary behavior with two years of exercise." In fact, participants who had worked out at least four days a week with a regimen of weight training, balance work, and yoga had healthier hearts and arteries and were fitter. The researchers said, "Literally any exercise is better than none."[44]

A 2019 study in the *American Journal of Epidemiology* found that "replacing just 30 minutes of sitting with any kind of movement, every day, could help" people have a longer life. The study reported that "getting up for half an hour of light activity—like walking, when a person would usually be sitting—corresponded to an estimated 17% lower risk of early death." The study also found that "the same amount of moderate or vigorous exercise corresponded to about a 35% lower mortality risk."[45]

Many folks our age remember and love the actor Dick Van Dyke. You may want to consider his newest book, *Keep Moving*. Dick exercises five days per week at age 91 and can show you how to do the same. He has a fun and folksy way to encourage you to "keep moving every day like there's no tomorrow."[46]

Who and Where

We encourage you to find a walking partner (which could also include a pet) and a safe place to walk. Some people find walking is conducive to thinking and chatting. A partner also makes every walk a bit safer. A safe place to walk is also requisite. Safety not only means safe from people, but vehicles also. With more people driving while distracted, keep your distance from vehicles.

Many folks don't seem to know or abide by the traffic rules for bicycles, and cyclists often ride on sidewalks. This can be dangerous for the walkers and the cyclists, so be on alert. Cornell University says, "As a general rule of thumb, it's not a good idea to encourage bicycling on sidewalks…The problem is that…bicyclists are not safer on the sidewalk."[47]

The great thinker and poet Henry David Thoreau wrote, "An early-morning walk is a blessing for the whole day."[48] So get out early, keep it simple, walk as much, and as often, as you can. Walking is great for your body, so take a walk today. Get off your butt—it's killing you!

13

FLEXIBILITY–MORE IMPORTANT THAN EVER

One of the biggest issues for all of us as we age is the loss of flexibility, or *range of motion* (ROM). Reduced ROM can cause problems ranging from inconvenience to injuries. The accumulation, over the years, of injuries to our joints may keep us from doing things we could easily do when we were younger. The shortening of muscles, ligaments, and tendons, mostly from disuse, reduces our ROM. With aging, our muscles lose strength and elasticity. For example, low-back flexibility is important, with an estimated 80 percent of US citizens experiencing low-back pain at some point, and it is the second leading cause of disability.[1]

SilverSneakers.com contributor Nicholas White says, "Ultimately, flexibility is about enjoying your life. By increasing your range of motion, you'll be less prone to injury while exercising, traveling, or playing with your grandkids. You'll feel less stiff and more comfortable in everyday activities like walking, lifting, bending, and even driving. You'll improve your posture, circulation, and balance while relieving pain and stress."[2] What's not to like about that?

Phil discovered that when his front upper-leg muscles weren't flexible enough, with all the running he was doing, his kneecap wouldn't properly track in the groove on the femur in which it glides. He would stretch his quadriceps muscle group, and the problem would disappear. On the other hand, Phil's wife, Brenda, had *great* flexibility, so when she had a similar kneecap problem, instead of stretching she went on a muscle strengthening program, which gave her relief because the stronger muscles better stabilized her kneecaps. One thing to keep in mind is that strength and flexibility need to be balanced. Too much of one without enough the other can lead to problems.

Most of us over 50 years of age need improved strength and flexibility. The good news is, stretching is one aspect of fitness that can be done almost any time and anywhere. You just need to remember to do it. According to Mayo Clinic, "Stretching and flexibility may take a back seat to your exercise routine. The main concern is exercising, not stretching, right? Not so fast. Stretching [and better flexibility] may help you:

- improve your performance in physical activities;

- decrease your risk of injuries;

- help your joints move through their full range of motion; and

- enable your muscles to work most effectively."[3]

Stretching to Improve Range of Motion (ROM)

Improving our ROM is not too complicated. We recommend *static stretching* as an effective way to improve ROM and improve the circulation of blood to our muscles. We recommend stretching your major muscle groups between two and three times weekly. When you perform a static stretch, you want to gradually elongate the muscle, hold the elongated position, and then let the muscle return to its resting position. Gradually work toward holding the stretch for 30 seconds in the elongated position. In problem areas, you may hold for 60 seconds.

For example, if we want to improve the ROM of our low back and hamstrings (muscles on the back of the upper leg), you can slowly and gently bend forward and let gravity stretch the back and legs. *Do not* continue if you have sharp pain. If you merely feel the stretch and have no pain, you should hold that position for 30 to 60 seconds.

If your front leg muscles need stretching, just put your right ankle up on your left thigh. Now put your right hand on your right knee and push gently. Just the weight of your hand may be enough. You want to feel stretch in your right thigh, but not pain. If you have pain, stop! Gradually, with repetitions the right knee will move down toward the floor more readily. Now repeat with the left leg. Over time, your range of motion will increase. Concentrate your stretches on major muscle groups such as your calves, thighs, hips, lower back, neck, and shoulders. Make sure you stretch both sides. Also stretch muscles and joints you routinely use. Don't bounce. Stretch in a smooth movement. Bouncing as you stretch can injure your muscles.

If you have been inactive (sedentary) and have access to a pool, you may want to stretch and exercise in the water. Exercising in water supports your joints and allows freedom of movement. You can either perform water exercises on your own or in a class.[4] Others find that exercise that combines both mental and physical discipline, such as yoga or tai chi, which use a series of body poses, can help to increase balance, strength, and flexibility. You can also find nice infographics, videos, and free resources on flexibility and stretching exercises online at Go4Life (from the National Institute of Aging) at tinyurl .com/yb7dbs6v.

The good news with stretching is that, in the absence of pain, it's hard to overdo stretching training. Although one can become too flexible, this is seldom a problem for us over the age of 50. Know yourself!

14

LIFTING WEIGHTS IS NOT JUST FOR ATHLETES

Many folks are intimidated about going to the gym because of the muscular people they encounter. But older Americans stand to gain the most from weight lifting of any segment of our society. Researchers have found at least ten benefits to strength training as we age:[1]

1. Improved functional strength and flexibility, making us less vulnerable to falls or other injuries.

2. Increased bone mass and density help protect us against osteoporosis (thinning of our bones), which helps prevent fractures.

3. Increased muscle strength. Each decade after the age of 30, we lose 3 to 5 percent of our muscle mass, which weakens us.

4. Lower body fat and a more favorable body composition. A gain in muscle may cause your body weight to stay the same despite fat loss; but this is still better for your health.

5. Reduced resting blood pressure.

6. Reduced low-back pain. Strength training can increase low-back strength and prevent or alleviate low-back pain.

7. Reduced pain of arthritis.

8. Reduced symptoms of other chronic diseases such as depression, heart disease, type 2 diabetes, and sleep disorders.

9. Enhanced appearance, self-confidence, and self-esteem.

10. Increased serotonin, the "feel good" hormone, resulting in better moods.

The American College of Sports Medicine recommends lifting light weight at moderate intensity twice a week for anyone 50 and older.[2] A regular program of strength training, combined with aerobic exercises, can help reduce, or prevent, many functional declines associated with growing older.

Even more impressive are the results of a recent study of more than 80,000 adults led by the University of Sydney that concluded, "Light weight lifting, push-ups, and sit-ups could add years to your life." It is the "largest study to compare the mortality outcomes of different types of exercise and reported that people who did strength-based exercise had a 23-percent reduction in risk of premature death by any means and a 31-percent reduction in cancer-related death."[3]

How to Get Started

A lot of choices are available. The most effective approach is to join a gym that can offer you a variety of training choices and a professional staff to educate and guide you. Here are options in the order we recommend them:

1. *Machines.* Strength training machines use weights (most often) but also can use rubber bands, springs, air cylinders, or even flexible rods to supply resistance. Generally, these machines are safer than free weights.

2. *Body weight lifting.* These are calisthenics—push-ups, pull-ups, dips, wall-sits, lunges, and bent-knee sit-ups. They can be done with little equipment and reduce opportunities for injury. Classes such as Pilates, Jazzercise, HIIT (high intensity interval training), CrossFit, and the like can be helpful for aerobic and muscle fitness.

3. *Free weights.* These are the most likely to result in an injury

if not done properly. Free weights come in a variety of styles, including barbells, dumbbells, and kettlebells.

You can find a description of weight lifting and strength training moves online and in many other sources. The CDC has a free booklet, *Growing Stronger: Strength Training for Older Adults*, which we recommend.[4] But starting with a personal trainer is wise to avoid beginner mistakes and injury risk.

How often you will do strength training depends on what works for you. In most cases older folks should work a muscle twice a week, with 72 hours between workouts of that muscle. In Phil's lab they found that few lifters of any age can repeat working a muscle group within 48 hours, and that older lifters take a bit longer to recover. So if you lift on Monday, don't work that muscle group again before Thursday. Repeat the next Monday and Thursday.

You can choose lifts depending on how often you work out. If you can lift every day, then on Monday you can do one-third of your lifts (upper body/arms, core/trunk, or lower body/legs), the second third on Tuesday, and the remaining third on Wednesday. Thursday you repeat Monday's workout, etc., and take Sunday off.

What to Expect?

About 24 hours after your first weight training session you may be sore. This is a *good* thing. It should not be unbearably painful, but a little soreness is assurance you accomplished something. The pain will peak at 48 hours and then resolve quickly. It's better to start off easy and build up gradually, which will reduce this problem and give you better results.

The first six to eight weeks you should notice a rapid increase in your training capacity. Your muscles and your nervous system are essentially learning how to lift weights. After that the rate of increase may be slower. Also, as you are starting out, you may want to eat more protein. According to a 2018 research review, "Eating more protein (while weight lifting) can significantly augment the effects of lifting weights, especially for people past the age of 40."[5]

So What?

For all older adults, a regular program of strengthening and aerobic exercises can help prevent, reduce, or even reverse many of the functional declines associated with aging. You can be one of those people if you will begin strength training and keep it up. It's a lifelong lifestyle change. You can do it!

15

TIPS TO AVOID COLORECTAL CANCER

Excluding skin cancers, colorectal cancer (CRC) is the third most common cancer *and* the third leading cancer killer in men *and* women in the US. The ACS estimated there would be about 140,000 new cases of colorectal cancer (and about 51,000 deaths) in 2018. Sadly, many of those cancers and deaths could be avoided or even prevented.[1]

To Lower Your Risk of CRC

When it comes to CRC, the ACS says, "There are things you can do that might help lower your risk, such as changing the risk factors that you can control."[2] Here are some controllable factors:

Weight, Activity, Nutrition, and Family History[3]

- *Weight.* Being overweight, obese or having more belly fat (a larger waistline) increases risk of colorectal cancer. Obese women are 93 percent more likely to develop early onset colorectal cancer compared with those at normal weight, according to a study involving more than 85,000 women who were followed for 22 years.[4]

- *Physical activity.* Regular moderate activity lowers the risk, and vigorous activity might have greater benefit. A meta-analysis of 52 studies found that the most physically active individuals had a 24 percent lower risk of colon cancer than those who were the least physically active.[5]

• *Nutrition.* Diets high in vegetables, fruits, and whole grains (and low in red and processed meats) have been linked with lower rates of colorectal cancer. Some studies suggest that fiber in the diet, especially from whole grains, may lower the risk. Several studies have found a higher risk of colorectal cancer with increased alcohol intake, especially among men. Also, avoid excess alcohol.[6]

• *Family history.* If you have a family history of colorectal polyps or cancer, talk with your doctor about your risk, as additional screening may be necessary.

Not Smoking[7]

Long-term smoking increases the risk of colorectal cancer as well as many other cancers and health problems. Quitting smoking helps lower your risk.

Nonsteroidal Anti-Inflammatory Drugs (NSAIDs)[8]

Many studies have found that regularly taking aspirin or other NSAIDs, such as ibuprofen (Motrin, Advil) and naproxen (Aleve), have lower risk of colorectal cancer; however, NSAIDs can cause serious or even life-threatening side effects. Nevertheless, if your doctor has recommended a daily aspirin tablet for you, the ACS says it "may also have the added benefit of reducing the risk of colorectal cancer." But we emphasize that you should check with your doctor before starting aspirin on a regular basis.

Hormone Replacement Therapy for Women[9]

Taking estrogen and progesterone after menopause may reduce a woman's risk of developing colorectal cancer; however, they may cause significant side effects. The ACS says, these medicines are "not commonly recommended just to lower colorectal cancer risk. If you're considering using menopausal hormone therapy, be sure to discuss the pros and cons with your doctor." The USPSTF recommends against using HRT for chronic conditions and to lower cancer risk.[10] We do not recommend HRT for colon cancer prevention.

Herbs or Supplements

The NCMD tells health professionals, "Olive oil, magnesium, and garlic consumption may decrease the risk of colon cancer. Recommend that patients consider increasing garlic consumption and suggest they substitute olive oil for other oils they commonly use in their diet."[11] The NCMD rates dietary intake of olive oil, magnesium (in foods such as legumes, whole grains, vegetables [especially broccoli, squash, and green leafy vegetables], seeds, and nuts), and garlic as "likely safe" and "possibly effective" at preventing colon cancer.

To Prevent CRC

Lowering your risk of CRC is one thing, but avoiding or preventing CRC is a hundred times better! And the great news is that CRC can be prevented for most people.[12] The American College of Gastroenterology (ACG) says, "Colorectal cancer...affects men and women equally. Yet few Americans know that CRC can be prevented—not just detected—through colonoscopy. One in three adults—23 million Americans between 50 and 75 years old—is not getting tested for colorectal cancer as recommended."[13]

A large study of folks aged 50 to 90 years reported that people who failed to be up-to-date on CRC screening had a 2.6-times higher risk of dying from colorectal cancer compared to those who were up-to-date on screening. It's even worse for those who do not receive follow-up testing after an abnormal result—those people had about sevenfold higher risk of death from colorectal cancer.[14]

Without doubt, regular CRC screening is the most powerful solution for preventing colorectal cancer. CRC almost always starts in colon polyps (lumps that grow on the inside of the colon). It can take 10 to 15 years for them to develop into CRC. With regular screening, most polyps can be found and removed long before they become cancerous. As of 2018, the ACS changed its guidelines so that if you're age 45 or older, you should start getting screened for CRC;[15] while the USPSTF still recommends starting at age 50;[16] therefore, most insurance companies are not covering CRC screening for folks 45 to 50 years old. Nevertheless, it's critical for all our readers to have CRC screening, and it's covered by all insurance companies.

It's important to understand that CRC screening tests can be divided into cancer prevention and cancer detection tests. Cancer prevention tests have the potential to reveal images of both cancer and polyps, whereas cancer detection tests typically help detect cancer but not precancerous polyps. ACG recommends that cancer prevention tests should be offered first, and the preferred CRC prevention test is colonoscopy every 10 years, beginning at age 45. They say cancer detection tests "should be offered to patients who decline colonoscopy or another cancer prevention test."[17]

ACS says, "Several test options are available for colorectal cancer screening. There are some differences among the tests to consider, but the most important thing is to get screened, no matter which test you choose." The Affordable Care Act requires both private insurers and Medicare to cover the costs of CRC screening tests, because these tests are recommended by the USPSTF.[18] Test options include:

- Stool-based tests (cancer detection tests), of which there are several. However, as of our writing, the most heavily advertised test (to physicians and consumers) is Cologuard (a DNA [deoxyribonucleic acid] test). The FDA says, "Cologuard is indicated to screen adults of either sex, 50 years or older, who are at typical average-risk for CRC. A positive result may indicate the presence of CRC or advanced adenoma and should be followed by diagnostic colonoscopy. Cologuard is not a replacement for diagnostic colonoscopy or surveillance colonoscopy in high-risk individuals." Cologuard is an option for those not willing or able to have a colonoscopy, which many experts still considered the first choice. More information from the FDA about this test can be found at tinyurl.com/y72tl385.

- Visual exams (cancer prevention tests), of which there are several. The most performed and recommended is colonoscopy every ten years. It has become the gold standard for CRC screening and prevention, but it's no one's idea of a pleasant day. Preparations the day before are inconvenient, and you must adjust your diet and medications. Frequent trips to the bathroom the day before the test are part of the process, and while anesthesia makes the test painless, anesthesia requires significant pre- and post-test rituals and costs. As a result, many people who should be screened fail to do so. For people who feel colonoscopy is too expensive or too much trouble, an option like Cologard makes CRC screening possible.

ACS emphasizes it's important that everyone talk to their health-care professional about which tests might be good options and to check insurance coverage for your copay for each test option. Senior news editor for cancer.org, Stacy Simon, says, "The guidelines stress that these screening tests must be repeated at regular intervals to be effective. And, if you choose to be screened with a test other than colonoscopy, any abnormal test result must be followed up with a colonoscopy to complete the screening process."[19]

No matter which test you choose, the most effective way to prevent CRC is to get screened regularly. As a result of CRC screening, this cancer has been prevented in millions, and more than one million folks in the US today are survivors of colorectal cancer.[20]

16

AVOID
MENOPAUSE MISERY

Menopause is when a woman's menstrual periods permanently end. It happens as a woman ages because her ovaries make fewer of the female hormones (estrogen and progesterone) that regulate the menstrual cycle. Menopause normally occurs from age 40 to age 59 (average age 51) and is a gradual process that can take a number of years. *Surgical menopause* occurs when a woman's ovaries are surgically removed before menopause. *Perimenopause* is the term for the three to five years before a woman has her final period and enters menopause.[1]

The most bothersome symptoms of menopause are vasomotor symptoms (VMS), primarily consisting of hot flashes, night sweats, and flushes, as well as the genitourinary syndrome of menopause (GSM), primarily resulting in vaginal dryness, burning, and irritation, as well as painful intercourse. Other symptoms include "brain fog," headaches, trouble sleeping, tiredness, sadness, anxiety, mood swings, and weight gain.

There isn't a set treatment for menopause. As a result, there are many ways to manage the symptoms of menopause that should be discussed with your healthcare professional. But let's discuss a few recommended options.

Nonhormonal Therapies

For recommended therapies, in a 2015 statement, the North American Menopause Society (NAMS) concluded, "Cognitive-behavioral therapy and, to a lesser extent, clinical hypnosis have been shown to be effective in reducing VMS. Paroxetine (Brisdelle) is the only nonhormonal medication approved by the FDA for the management of VMS, although other prescription medications (including selective serotonin reuptake inhibitors [SSRIs, of which paroxetine is one], selective norepinephrine reuptake inhibitors [SNRIs], gabapentinoids [i.e. gabapentin], and clonidine) show evidence of efficacy."[2]

Under the heading "Recommend with caution," they say, "Some therapies that may be beneficial for alleviating VMS are weight loss, mindfulness-based stress reduction...[and] soy isoflavones."[3]

Their "Do not recommend at this time" categories include "cooling techniques, avoidance of triggers, exercise, yoga, paced respiration, relaxation, over-the-counter supplements and herbal therapies, acupuncture, calibration of neural oscillations, and chiropractic interventions." As to these therapies, NAMS says, "There are negative, insufficient, or inconclusive data suggesting [that these] should not be recommended for managing VMS."[4]

Dietary Supplements

The NMCD suggests, "Due to the concern about the safety of [hormone therapies], many more women are turning to phytoestrogens and other natural products for menopausal symptoms." They tell doctors, "Explain to women that natural medicines with estrogenic effects might not be any safer than conventional estrogenic drugs. At this point, there is not enough data from large-scale clinical trials to compare safety of phytoestrogens with conventional estrogen products."[5]

NMCD agrees with NAMS and adds, "Soy has the most evidence for effectiveness and some women might benefit from taking it. Soy protein–containing foods are preferred over soy extract supplements which have concentrated isoflavones. There is less known about the long-term safety of soy extract supplements."[6] NMCD says, "Black cohosh might also help some women. Due to concerns about potential liver damage, women taking black cohosh should consider getting liver function tests."[7] NMCD instructs doctors, "Explain to women that these supplements are not 'big guns.' They seem to provide only modest relief, if any."[8]

Finally, NMCD tells women not to waste their money on "red clover, DHEA, flaxseed, chasteberry, kudzu, alfalfa, hops, licorice, evening primrose oil, Panax ginseng, wild yam, or vitamin E." They say, "There's not enough evidence these are beneficial. Steer patients away from dong quai due to potential safety concerns."[9]

If you are going to take a dietary supplement for menopausal symptoms, we strongly suggest you view (if available) or purchase the "Menopause Supplements Review" from ConsumerLab.com at tinyurl.com/yc6to2ke.

Menopausal Hormone Therapy

Prescribing hormone therapy before menopause (for birth control) and after menopause (for menopause symptom control, colon cancer risk reduction, and osteoporosis risk reduction) has been controversial. As of 2018, here are the ACS recommendations:[10]

- Before menopause, consider nonhormonal forms of birth control (such as modern natural family planning) because birth control methods that use hormones might increase breast cancer risk.

- After menopause, many women are given hormone therapy with estrogen (often combined with progesterone) to help relieve symptoms of menopause and help prevent osteoporosis (thinning of the bones). There are two main types of hormone therapy: (1) For women who still have a uterus, doctors generally prescribe estrogen and progesterone (called *combined hormone therapy* or *HT*). Progesterone is needed because estrogen alone can increase the risk of cancer of the uterus. (2) For women who've had a hysterectomy (who no longer have a uterus), estrogen alone can be used. This is called *estrogen therapy* (ET).

  » HT after menopause increases the risk of breast cancer, the chances of dying from breast cancer, and the likelihood that the cancer may be found at a more advanced stage. However, the increased risk is only in current and recent users. A woman's breast cancer risk returns to that of the general population within five years of stopping treatment.

» Although many alternative or complimentary practitioners sell *bioidentical HT* as safer, the ACS says, "The use of bioidentical hormones should be considered to have the same health risks as any other type of hormone therapy."[11] NAMS says, "Compounded bioidentical HT should be avoided, given concerns about safety, including the possibility of overdosing or underdosing, lack of efficacy and safety studies, and lack of a label providing risks."[12]

» ET does not seem to increase the risk of breast cancer much, if at all, unless used long term (i.e., for more than 15 years) where it has been found to increase the risk of ovarian and breast cancer.

As of 2017, here are the recommendations of the NAMS:[13]

- Hormone therapy (HT) remains the most effective treatment for VMS and GSM and has been shown to prevent bone loss and fracture.

- The risks of HT differ depending on type, dose, duration of use, route of administration, timing of initiation, and whether a progestogen is used. Treatment should be individualized to identify the most appropriate HT...using the best available evidence to maximize benefits and minimize risks, with periodic reevaluation of the benefits and risks of continuing or discontinuing HT.

- For women aged younger than 60 years or who are within 10 years of menopause onset and have no contraindications, the benefit-risk ratio is most favorable for treatment of bothersome VMS and for those at elevated risk for bone loss or fracture. For women who initiate HT more than 10 or 20 years from menopause onset, or are aged 60 years or older, the benefit-risk ratio appears less favorable because of the greater absolute risks of coronary heart disease, stroke, venous thromboembolism (blood clots), and dementia.

- For bothersome GSM symptoms not relieved with over-the-counter therapies and without indications for use of systemic HT, low-dose vaginal estrogen therapy or other therapies are recommended.

The HT story remains complex and controversial. The ACS advises:[14]

> Along with the increased risk of breast cancer, HT also appears to increase the risk of heart disease, blood clots, and strokes. It does lower the risk of colorectal cancer and osteoporosis, but this must be weighed against the possible harms, especially since there are other ways to prevent and treat osteoporosis, and screening can sometimes prevent colon cancer. ET (estrogen therapy) does not seem to increase breast cancer risk, but it does increase the risk of stroke.

> At this time there aren't many strong reasons to use postmenopausal HT or ET other than possibly for the short-term relief of menopausal symptoms. The decision to use HT should be made by a woman and her doctor after weighing the possible risks and benefits, including the severity of her menopausal symptoms, and considering her other risk factors for heart disease, breast cancer, and osteoporosis. If they decide she should try HT for symptoms of menopause, it's usually best to use it at the lowest dose that works for her and for as short a time as possible.

Hormone therapy has potential benefits and risks, not to mention significant costs. Before starting any menopause therapy, invest first in a significant discussion with your physician.

17

SLEEP SOUNDER

Tim Herrera, the Smarter Living editor for the *New York Times*, writes, "Imagine this: Someone walks up to you and pitches you on a brand new, magical pill. This pill can measurably improve your memory, overall cognitive performance, ability to learn new information, receptivity to facial cues, mood, ability to handle problems, metabolism, risk for heart disease and immune system. Would you buy it?" He answers, "Yeah, yeah, you saw this coming: That pill exists, but not in pill form. You can have all of those benefits for free, and all it takes is going to bed a little bit earlier. That's it."[1] And he's right! Let us explain why.

As we age, changes to our sleep patterns are normal. We tend to have a harder time falling asleep and more trouble staying asleep than when we were younger. The National Sleep Foundation (NSF) writes, "Studies on the sleep habits of older Americans show an increase in the time it takes to fall asleep...[and an increase in] waking up during the night."[2]

Not getting enough sleep may be harmful to your health. According to British experts at the NHS:[3]

1. *Sleep boosts immunity.* If you seem to catch every cold and flu that's going around, your bedtime could be to blame. A 2019 study from Germany showed restful sleep strengthens the potency of certain immune cells and improves their chances of attaching to—and eventually destroying—cells infected with viruses.[4]

2. *Sleep can slim you.* Sleeping less may mean you put on weight! Studies have shown that people who sleep less than seven hours a day tend to gain more weight and have a higher risk of becoming obese than those who get seven hours of slumber. Other research shows if you don't get enough sleep, it's harder to lose excess weight and keep it off.[5] The NHS says, "It's believed to be because sleep-deprived people have reduced levels of leptin [the chemical that makes you feel full] and increased levels of ghrelin [the hunger-stimulating hormone]."

3. *Sleep boosts mental well-being.* Given that a single sleepless night can make you irritable and moody the following day, it's not surprising that chronic sleep debt may lead to long-term mood disorders such as depression and anxiety. When people with anxiety or depression were surveyed to calculate their sleeping habits, it turned out that most of them slept for less than six hours a night. A 2018 study found, "A sleepless night can leave the brain spinning with anxiety the next day." The researchers concluded, "People with anxiety disorders often have trouble sleeping. The new results uncover the reverse effect—that poor sleep can induce anxiety." They add, "After sleep deprivation, anxiety levels in these healthy people were 30 percent higher than when they had slept. On average, the anxiety scores reached levels seen in people with anxiety disorders."[6]

4. *Sleep reduces the risk of diabetes.* Studies have suggested that people who usually sleep less than five hours a night have an increased risk of developing diabetes. It seems that missing out on deep sleep may lead to type 2 diabetes by changing the way the body processes glucose, which the body uses for energy.

5. *Sleep increases sex drive.* Men and women who don't get enough quality sleep have lower libidos and less of an interest in sex, research suggests. Men who suffer from

sleep apnea—a disorder in which breathing difficulties lead to interrupted sleep—also tend to have lower testosterone levels, which can lower libido.

6. *Sleep wards off heart disease.* Long-standing sleep deprivation seems to be associated with increased heart rate, an increase in blood pressure, and higher levels of certain chemicals linked with inflammation, which may put extra strain on your heart—and your arteries. A 2019 study from Spain found that "sleeping fewer than six hours a night or waking frequently raises your risk of developing damaging plaque in arteries throughout your body, not just your heart."[7] US researchers found "sleeping too little increases your risk of heart attack or stroke. Those who slept seven to eight hours a night had the lowest heart risk on average."[8]

A 2018 first-of-its-kind study of almost 400,000 American adults in all 50 states and DC found, "One-third of US adults say they sleep less than six hours a night, which is 15 percent more than…15 years ago"[9] and 30 percent less than in 1910, when folks slept an average of nine hours per night.[10] The CDC reports, "Eighty percent of people report sleep problems at least once per week. That results in 1.23 million lost days of work per year and $400 billion in economic losses annually."[11] Lack of sleep is so bad that in 2017 the CDC "called *insufficient sleep a public health epidemic*."[12]

The University of Michigan National Poll on Healthy Aging reported that "in a typical week, nearly half of older adults (46%) reported that they regularly have trouble falling asleep: 32% on 1-2 nights a week and 15% on three or more nights. Older adults who described their health as fair or poor were more likely to report trouble falling asleep…Over a third of older adults (36%) reported using some type of medication to help with sleep including prescription sleep medications, over-the-counter (OTC) medications promoted as night-time formulations, herbal/natural sleep aids (like melatonin) or prescription pain medications."[13]

It is a myth that sleep requirements decline with age. According to the National Sleep Foundation (NSF), "Research demonstrates that our sleep needs remain constant throughout adulthood."[14] However, *insomnia*, meaning "difficulty falling asleep or staying asleep," is more common among older adults. According to NSF's Sleep in America poll, 44 percent of older persons experience one or more of the symptoms of insomnia at least a few nights per week. Insomnia may be acute (lasting a few days or weeks), or chronic (lasting more than one month). Insomnia is often related to an underlying medical or emotional condition or the medications used to treat them.[15]

Generally, adults need seven to nine hours of sleep each night to restore their mental and physical state. A Gallup poll from 2013 states, "Americans currently average 6.8 hours of sleep at night, down more than an hour from 1942."[16] The *Wall Street Journal* reported, "Some studies have even suggested that, if you go through a workweek while consistently sleep-deprived, you will finish the week with 15 fewer IQ points than you began it with."[17] Other research, commissioned by fitness app Freeletics, looked at the specific reasons people gave for experiencing a bad day and found not getting enough sleep was the biggest contributing factor—and the average American admits to having an average of 60 bad days a year![18]

So what's keeping seniors awake? According to the National Sleep Foundation, there are a number of potential issues:[19]

- As we age, our circadian rhythms (brain signals that coordinate the timing of our bodily functions, including sleep) change. "Older people tend to become sleepier earlier in the evening and wake earlier in the morning compared to younger adults. This pattern is called *advanced sleep phase syndrome*."[20] The sleep rhythm is shifted forward so that seven or eight hours of sleep are still obtained but the individuals will wake up earlier because they have gone to sleep early.

- Other common problems causing sleep disturbances include snoring, obstructive sleep apnea (OSA), restless leg syndrome (RLS), and depression or anxiety. Untreated

OSA can put you at risk for cardiovascular disease, headaches, memory loss (including dementia and Alzheimer's), and depression. It's simple to diagnose with a sleep study and can be effectively treated. The Cleveland Clinic has a nice handout on "Sleep Disorders in Older Adults" at tinyurl.com/y73lr7hp.

- You may experience sleep-disturbing medical problems such as menopause and its hot flashes, prostate enlargement and the resultant need to urinate more frequently, arthritis and the nighttime discomfort it can cause in certain positions, and gastroesophageal reflux disease and the heartburn it causes when lying flat. All increase with age.

- Many other medical conditions (diabetes, renal failure, respiratory diseases, Parkinson's, multiple sclerosis, immune disorders, and others) are associated with sleep problems and disorders. If you're wrestling with poor sleep, you may want to see your doctor or a sleep specialist for an evaluation.

NSF recommends, "In order to wake up feeling refreshed, it's important to focus on both sleep quantity—how much sleep we get each night—as well as sleep quality, which indicates how well we sleep. Poor sleep quality can cause us to feel groggy the next day and may even be linked to an increased risk of Alzheimer's disease. But determining the quality of your sleep is less straightforward than counting the number of hours you get. Learn the signs of poor sleep quality and discover how to improve it."[21]

So, step one is figure out your divine design. How much sleep do you really need? Of course, if you always wake up fatigued, you may not be getting enough restful sleep. But a particular number, such as eight hours a night, may not be right for you. The "right amount" is the amount you need to wake up refreshed, rested, and energized the next morning. For my patients, I suggest they keep a sleep diary. NSF has a great one at tinyurl.com/yy5x4f26.

Once you're getting the right number of hours of sleep, look over this list from the NSF to see if you have any of these signs that your sleep quality needs to improve:[22]

- It takes you more than 30 minutes to fall asleep after getting into bed.
- You regularly wake up more than once per night.
- You find yourself staying awake for more than 20 minutes after waking up in the middle of the night.
- You spend less than 85 percent of your time in bed asleep.

If any of these are true for you, the NSF suggests these "sleep hygiene" steps to improve sleep quality:[23]

1. Stop watching television or using electronic devices such as a laptop or cell phone at least 30 minutes before bedtime. The blue light emitted from these gadgets can make it difficult to fall asleep.

2. Set your bedroom thermostat between 60- and 67-degrees Fahrenheit. Sleeping in a room that is either too warm or too cool interferes with your ability to drift off.

3. Follow a consistent sleep schedule. Having poor bedtime habits, such as going to bed too early (before you're tired) or too late (when you're overly tired) can make it more difficult to sleep soundly. A 2018 study found, "Adults who have a regular bedtime are likely to weigh less, have lower blood sugar and face a lower risk of heart disease and diabetes."[24] Also, research from Northwestern University and the University of Surrey in the United Kingdom suggests that self-described "night owls" have a 10 percent greater risk of death than "morning people" and that they have "higher risks for conditions such as diabetes or psychological disorders."[25] Benjamin Franklin recognized the health benefits of early rising and put this old proverb in the 1735 edition of his *Poor Richard's Almanack* [sic]:

"Early to bed and early to rise, makes a man healthy
wealthy and wise."[26]

4. Create a relaxing pre-bedtime routine, such as taking a bath
   or reading a book. Brushing one's teeth, putting on pajamas,
   and turning off the lights can be signals to the body that it's
   time to secrete melatonin, the hormone that helps humans
   feel sleepy. One study showed people who regularly listened
   to music to fall asleep dozed off faster with music than
   without.[27] Engaging in high-energy or stressful activities
   lowers the odds of an easy transition to sleep.

5. Limit your alcohol consumption to one (women) or two
   (men) drinks per day because alcohol can disturb sleep.

6. Avoid caffeinated beverages within four to six hours of
   bedtime, and alcohol within three hours of going to bed.
   Some elderly folks may need to avoid these products up to
   eight hours before bedtime.

The CDC adds these suggestions:[28]

1. Be consistent. Get up at the same time each morning,
   including on the weekends.

2. Make sure your bedroom is quiet, dark, and relaxing.

3. Remove electronic devices, such as TVs, computers, and
   smart phones, from the bedroom.

4. Avoid large meals before bedtime.

5. Exercise. Being physically active during the day, but well
   before bedtime, can help you fall asleep more easily at night.

We have a couple of other tips for you to consider. A study in the
Journal of Experimental Psychology said, "Bedtime worry, including worrying about incomplete future tasks, is a significant contributor to difficulty falling asleep. Previous research showed that writing about one's
worries can help individuals fall asleep." This study concluded, "To
facilitate falling asleep, individuals may derive benefit from writing a

very specific to-do list for five [minutes] at bedtime." They also found, "The more specifically participants wrote their to-do list [the longer and more specific their to-do lists], the faster they subsequently fell asleep."[29]

This is related to the research that shows that writing down worries can stop worrying that can wake you during the night, reduce stress levels, strengthen your memory, and eliminate distractions.[30]

Another recent small study reported that woolly flannel pajamas might actually help sleep, possibly by better regulating body temperature. Earth.com writer Kyla Cathey reported the findings of a pair of studies in the journal *Nature and Science of Sleep*: "Participants wearing wool fell asleep about four minutes faster and enjoyed an average of seven minutes more sleep than their cotton-wearing counterparts… Seniors in merino flannel pajamas fell asleep in about 12 minutes, compared to 22 minutes for the polyester-wearers and 27 minutes for those in cotton."[31] Although a study back in 2004 found that only 34 percent of Americans wore pajamas, while 23 percent go with a shorts/T-shirt combo, and 22 percent wear only their birthday suit.[32]

Last, but far from least, is the fact that improving your spiritual health may improve your sleep. Researchers in 2019 reported that "those who believe in salvation and feel they have an unshakable relationship with God tend to sleep longer, fall asleep faster, and feel more rested in the morning."[33] One of the researchers said, "It makes intuitive sense. People who believe they're secure to God and will go to heaven when they die rest assured."[34] The study authors add:

> Regular churchgoers may experience less agitation in the wake of negative life events, and, ultimately, better quality sleep…However, one doesn't necessarily need a religious community to reduce stress. A nonorganizational religious practice, such as frequent reading of Scripture and prayer, can also reduce stress and facilitate sound sleep so long as the individual feels secure in the attachment to God and the person's place in the afterlife.

> Believers may be unable to comprehend why misfortune has befallen them, but they may nevertheless sleep better at night knowing that the universe is under the watchful eye

of a deity who, at the end of the day, remains deeply concerned with the well-being of the world and its inhabitants.[35]

Psychological and behavioral interventions are considered first-line treatments for insomnia. Guidelines from the American College of Physicians and the American Academy of Sleep Medicine recommend a therapy called *cognitive behavioral therapy* (CBT) as the first-line treatment for all adults with chronic insomnia disorder.[36] Nothing has been shown more effective for chronic sleep problems than what can be provided by a qualified Christian counselor or therapist.

Reuters reported on research finding that "people with insomnia who receive a digitized [app-based] version of cognitive behavioral therapy (CBT) as part of their treatment may find more symptom relief than those who only receive tips to improve their sleep routines."[37] Information on this new program can be found at tinyurl.com/y4xon293.

It's important to know that most of the prescriptions your doctor could write for insomnia should not be used for more than a few days or weeks and may be associated, at least with long-term use, with head injuries, cancer, and dementia.[38]

Melatonin is a popular supplement for sleep. Studies show it can help you fall asleep faster. The NMCD concludes, "Melatonin…might be worth a trial run for people with insomnia, particularly elderly patients."[39] They suggest a dose of 0.3 to 5 milligrams per day, saying, "Immediate-release melatonin is best for people with difficulty falling asleep, while sustained-release melatonin is better for people having trouble staying asleep."[40] Valerian is another supplement used as a sleep aid. NMCD tells us doctors, "Valerian is promising, but there's still not enough solid evidence to recommend it for most patients. If a patient wants to try it, don't worry too much."[41]

If you try these suggestions and still feel the quality of your sleep needs improvement, talk to your PCP, who can recommend lifestyle changes, medication, or other therapies that may improve how well you sleep. Or, if your spiritual health needs a checkup, consider seeing a pastoral professional or Christian counselor.

18

PROTECT YOUR SKIN

Skin cancer is by far the most common type of cancer according to the ACS.[1] Although there are many types of skin cancer, the big three are as described by the American Academy of Dermatology (AAD):[2]

1. Basal cell carcinoma (BCC) is the most common type of skin cancer.

   - BCCs frequently develop in people who have fair skin, yet they can occur in people with darker skin.

   - BCCs look like a flesh-colored, pearl-like bump or a pinkish patch of skin and develop after years of frequent sun exposure or indoor tanning.

   - BCC is common on the head, neck, and arms, yet it can form anywhere on the body, including the chest, abdomen, and legs.

2. Squamous-cell carcinoma (SCC) is the second most common type of skin cancer.

   - SCC is more common in light-skinned as opposed darker-skinned people.

   - SCC often looks like a red firm bump, scaly patch, or a sore that heals and then reopens.

   - SCC tends to form on skin that gets frequent sun

exposure, such as the rim of the ear, face, neck, arms, chest, and back.

3. Melanoma is the deadliest form of skin cancer.

- Melanoma frequently develops in a mole or suddenly appears as a new dark spot on the skin.

- Knowing the ABCDE warning signs of melanoma can help you find an early melanoma:[3]

  » A = Asymmetry—one half is unlike the other half.

  » B = Border—an irregular, scalloped or poorly defined border.

  » C = Color—is varied from one area to another; has shades of tan, brown or black, or is sometimes white, red, or blue.

  » D = Diameter—melanomas are usually greater than 6mm (the size of a pencil eraser) when diagnosed, but they can be smaller.

  » E = Evolving—a mole or skin lesion that looks different from the rest or is changing in size, shape, or color.

Skin cancers need to be discovered and treated early to prevent them from spreading into and damaging surrounding tissues or spreading around the body. The Skin Cancer Foundation recommends that you and your spouse do a head-to-toe examination of each other's skin every month so you can find any new or changing lesions that might be cancerous or precancerous.[4] Then, if you notice a spot on your skin that is different from others, or that changes, itches, or bleeds, make an appointment to see your healthcare professional or a dermatologist. Skin cancers are almost always curable when found and removed early. You can find a step-by-step guide to self-examination at tinyurl.com/y7aozlet.

Protecting your skin from harmful ultraviolet (UV) rays can reduce your risk of getting skin cancer, including melanoma. The US

Environmental Protection Agency estimates that the sun causes 90 percent of all nonmelanoma skin cancers, and other research links it to 65 percent of all melanomas.[5] The CDC says you can reduce your risk of skin damage and skin cancer using simple sun protection tips. This is important to know because the sun's ultraviolet (UV) rays can damage your skin in as little as 15 minutes. Follow these recommendations from the CDC to help protect yourself and your family:[6]

- *Shade.* Even though seeking shade under an umbrella, tree, or other shelter gives relief from the sun, your best bet to protect your skin is to use sunscreen or wear protective clothing when you're outside—even when you're in the shade.

- *Clothing.* When possible, wear long-sleeved shirts and long pants and skirts, which can provide protection from UV rays. Clothes made from tightly woven fabric offer the best protection. A wet T-shirt offers much less UV protection than a dry one, and darker colors may offer more protection than lighter colors. Some clothing certified under international standards comes with information on its ultraviolet protection factor. Keep in mind that a typical T-shirt has a sun protection factor (SPF) rating lower than 15, so use other types of protection as well.

- *Hat.* For the most protection, wear a hat with a brim all the way around that shades your face, ears, and the back of your neck. A tightly woven fabric, such as canvas, works best to protect your skin from UV rays. Avoid straw hats with holes that let sunlight through. A darker hat may offer more UV protection. And, if you wear a baseball cap, you should also protect your ears and the back of your neck by wearing clothing that covers those areas, using a broad-spectrum sunscreen with at least SPF 15.

- *Sunglasses.* Sunglasses can protect your eyes from UV rays and reduce the risk of cataracts. They also protect the tender skin around your eyes from sun exposure. Sunglasses that block both UVA and UVB rays offer the best protection. Most sunglasses sold in the US, regardless of cost, meet this standard. Wrap-around sunglasses work best because they block UV rays from sneaking in from the side.

- *Sunscreen.* Each product is assigned an SPF number that rates its effectiveness in blocking UV rays. Higher numbers indicate more protection. Always put on broad-spectrum sunscreen with at least an SPF of 15 before you go outside, even on slightly cloudy or cool days. The AAD says, "Choose a sunscreen that has an SPF of 30 or higher, is water resistant, and provides broad-spectrum coverage, which means it protects you from UVA and UVB rays."[7] Don't forget to put a thick layer on all parts of exposed skin. Get help for hard-to-reach places like your back. And remember, sunscreen works best when combined with other options to prevent UV damage.

  » Sunscreen tips from the AAD:[8]

    – Most sunscreen products work by absorbing, reflecting, or scattering sunlight. They contain chemicals that interact with the skin to protect it from UV rays. All products do not have the same ingredients. If your skin reacts badly to one product, try another one or see a doctor.

    – It takes at least 15 minutes for your skin to absorb the sunscreen and protect you. If you wait until you are in the sun to apply sunscreen, your skin is unprotected and can burn. I tell folks in my practice to remember what I call the *20/20 Rule*: Use a broad-spectrum sunscreen with an SPF of 20 and apply it at least 20 minutes before going outside.

    – Sunscreen wears off. Put it on again if you stay out

in the sun for more than two hours and after swimming, sweating, or toweling off.

- Sunscreen without an expiration date has a shelf life of no more than three years, but its shelf life is shorter if it has been exposed to high temperatures.

People who get sunburned usually haven't used enough sunscreen, haven't reapplied it after being in the sun, or have used an expired product. Your skin is exposed to the sun's harmful UV rays every time you go outside, even on cloudy days and in the winter. So whether you are on vacation or taking a brisk fall walk in your neighborhood, remember to use sunscreen.

A study published in *JAMA Dermatology* found that fewer than half of the patients at a dermatology clinic knew the meaning of terms like "broad spectrum" and "SPF."[9] So the AAD has developed an information handout on understanding sunscreen lingo. You can find it at tinyurl.com/n3hjrgm.

Are tanning beds safe? We don't recommend them, nor do dermatologists. According the American Society for Dermatologic Surgery (ASDS), "Exposure to the ultraviolet light from tanning beds can impact the skin in a variety of ways—including wrinkles, sun spots or freckles. And for one in every five Americans, this exposure can lead to skin cancer. The use of tanning beds and sun lamps is hazardous because the UV radiation they deliver can damage your skin. Dermatologists highly recommend not using tanning beds and sun lamps. There is growing evidence they may increase your risk of developing melanoma."[10]

The ASDS says, ""There is no such thing as a healthy suntan. Any change in your natural skin color is a sign of skin damage. Evidence suggests tanning greatly increases your risk of developing skin cancer."[11] They add, "If you are seeking a tanned appearance, consider sunless tanning products" instead of UV light.[12]

I recommend to all my patients that they apply an unscented moisturizing cream with an SPF of at least 15 to their exposed skin each day before leaving home—every day of the year. "Every day to keep skin cancer away," I say. But not only that; you'll look younger. In fact, in one study, daily sunscreen use reduced the effects of aging on skin by nearly 25 percent.[13] The bottom line is that sunscreen protects the skin from harmful UV rays and helps prevent skin cancer, and it may also reduce premature wrinkles and benefit your beauty.

SPIRITUAL
HEALTH TIPS

19

12 STEPS FOR SPIRITUAL STRENGTH TRAINING

As we've discussed in multiple tips, without a deliberate effort to move, and exercise, and strengthen, and nourish our fleshly bodies, we become fat and out of shape, get sick more often, and die prematurely. If most of us were forced to compete in a race, we would be embarrassed and finish near last—if we finished at all. In the same way, ignoring our spiritual health makes us spiritually flabby with weak moral muscles and weakened characters.

Of course, the opposite is also true. If we improve our physical health, strength, flexibility, and nutrition, we live a life with the potential for greater quality and quantity. We become stronger, healthier, and more capable. And if we pursue spiritual nutrition and training, we are better able to resist temptation, and we are equipped to win spiritual warfare and resist Satan.

Spiritual strength training and *spiritual nutrition* refer to those regular spiritual practices that benefit our health and our lives—activities or disciplines that produce spiritual, physical, emotional, and relational health.

Pastor John Ortberg says, "Practices such as reading Scripture and praying are important—not because they prove how spiritual we are— but because God can use them to lead us into life."[1] Although the Bible has no comprehensive "spiritual training list" that followers of Jesus should practice, it does command us to do certain things regularly.

Our experience is that these disciplines produce abundant fruit.

Like all of our tips, the key is to start small and make new healthful habits one at a time. Here are a dozen to consider—some of which we've discussed in more depth, but we hope this review will be helpful:

1. *Read, study, memorize, and meditate on God's Word.* God's Word is the foundation of our lives. In the Scriptures, God reveals Himself and His will for us. If we want to know and enjoy God, the place to begin is God's Word—the most powerful and reliable way He speaks to us. (Joshua 1:8; Jeremiah 15:16; Psalms 1:1-2; 119:11-16; Romans 1:16; Ephesians 6:17; 2 Timothy 3:16; Hebrews 4:12)

2. *"Rejoice always, pray continually, give thanks in all circumstances; for this is God's will for you in Christ Jesus"* *(1 Thessalonians 5:16-18).* Each of these activities involves talking to God—throughout the day, every day. Another word for this is *prayer.* Think of these first two disciplines like spiritual breathing. We breathe in God's Word, and we speak out our prayers of confession, adoration, thanksgiving, and praise to Him. (Psalm 100:4; Romans 8:28; Philippians 4:6; Hebrews 4:16; 1 Peter 5:6-7)

3. *Give generously of your treasure, time, and talent.* "Remember this: Whoever sows sparingly will also reap sparingly, and whoever sows generously will also reap generously" (2 Corinthians 9:6). Research suggests those who give generously are happier,[2] healthier,[3] less stressed,[4] less anxious,[5] and live longer.[6] A 1944 newspaper column is credited with first observing: "You make a living by what you get. You make a life by what you give."[7] Giving blesses others and delights us. No wonder the Bible says, "Each of you should give what you have decided in your heart to give, not reluctantly or under compulsion, for God loves a cheerful giver. And God is able to bless you abundantly, so that in all things at all times, having all that you need, you will abound in every good work" (2 Corinthians 9:7-8).

(Proverbs 11:24; 19:17; Matthew 23:11; Mark 9:35; 10:43-44; Luke 6:38; Acts 20:35; Colossians 3:23-24; 1 Timothy 6:17-18; 1 Peter 4:10)

4. *Fast.* "When you fast, do not look gloomy like the hypocrites…[but] anoint your head and wash your face, that your fasting may not be seen by others but by your Father who is in secret. And your Father who sees in secret will reward you" (Matthew 6:16-18 ESV). (Exodus 34:28; Ezekiel 8:21-23; 2 Samuel 12:15-17; Isaiah 58:3-7; Joel 2:12-13; Daniel 9:3; 10:3; Esther 4:16; Nehemiah 1:4; Psalm 35:13-14; Luke 2:37; 4:2-4; Acts 13:2-3)

5. *Worship (celebrate) God.* Worship is experiencing God and responding to Him. This can occur in celebration with others and alone with God. In worship, we focus our minds and hearts on God and let our praise go up to Him. God commands we worship only Him (Exodus 20:3) and Jesus said, "God is spirit, and his worshipers must worship in the Spirit and in truth" (John 4:24). (1 Chronicles 16:11; Psalms 95:6; 99:5; 100:2-4; 118:4; Romans 12:1-2; 1 Corinthians 14:26; Ephesians 5:19-20; James 4:8)

6. *Fellowship (build community) with other followers of Jesus.* It was said of the early believers, "They devoted themselves to the apostles' teaching and to fellowship, to the breaking of bread and to prayer" (Acts 2:42) and we're reminded, "Let us consider how we may spur one another on toward love and good deeds, not giving up meeting together, as some are in the habit of doing, but encouraging one another" (Hebrews 10:24-25). (Matthew 4:10; 28:17; John 17:21; Acts 3:8)

7. *Seek and dispense forgiveness.* Unforgiveness and its associated toxic ABCs (anger, bitterness, and cynicism) are slow, lethal toxins that poison us from the inside out. Forgiveness improves physical, mental/emotional,

relational, *and* physical health. We "forgive to live" and we "forgive to be forgiven." Jesus taught, "If you hold anything against anyone, forgive them, so that your Father in heaven may forgive you your sins" (Mark 11:25). We can forgive much because we have been forgiven much!

8. *Practice solitude, silence, Sabbath, and simplicity.* Solitude and silence are more a state of mind and heart than they are a place of quiet and peace—and by definition silence requires you to turn off all electronic tools (computer, phone, e-mail, social media, etc.). Sabbath has to do with taking regular time to rest and worship. Simplicity is a declaration of war on materialism, and it reorients our lives, perspectives, and attitudes. (Genesis 2:3; Leviticus 23:3; Psalms 4:8; 127:2; Matthew 11:28)

9. *Practice confession.* Jim Dennison writes, "There has been only one perfect person in human history. For the rest of us, transparency when we fail is a vital step toward redemption. Scripture calls us to confess our sins to our Father (1 John 1:9) and to each other (James 5:16). And it promises: 'Whoever conceals his transgressions will not prosper, but he who confesses and forsakes them will obtain mercy' (Proverbs 28:13 ESV)."[8] Confession is the pathway to release, righteousness, restoration, and recovery. (Psalm 32:3-5; Proverbs 28:13; Acts 3:19)

10. *Be discipled/mentored and disciple/mentor others.* Pastor Andy Stanley wisely points out, "We each have a treasure chest full of life experiences that will die with us unless we become intentional about distributing our wealth. The value of your life is found when we share those experiences."[9] His sermon on mentoring is the best I've heard. You can watch or listen to it at tinyurl.com/ y8xqfzx8. In it he says, "If you are over 40, you have the opportunity and obligation to share what you've learned

with those coming behind you."[10] (Matthew 28:19-20; Acts 5:42; Philippians 4:9; 2 Timothy 2:2; Titus 2:3-5)

11. *Voluntarily submit humbly to God and those in authority over us.* We commit to willingly yield our will, mind, and body for God's purposes so we can better hear, receive, and obey His Word. When we humbly submit to those in authority giving moral direction, we are also submitting and serving our Lord! (Psalm 40:8; Micah 6:8; John 14:15; Ephesians 5:21; Romans 13:1-7; Philippians 2:1-8; Colossians 3:23-24; 1 Peter 2:13-18; 3:1)

12. *Pursue purity.* Practicing purity from "the deeds of the flesh" is a discipline because our natural inclinations draw us toward sexual and emotional impurity—toward immorality, idolatry, jealousy, greed, gluttony, gossiping. "The lust of the flesh, the lust of the eyes, and the pride of life comes not from the Father but from the world" (1 John 2:16). We must be disciplined to flee immorality and pursue pure thoughts and actions. (Exodus 20:14; Matthew 5:28-29; Colossians 3:5; 1 Corinthians 10:13; James 1:14-15)

The Bible teaches, "The one who says he resides in God ought himself to walk just as Jesus walked" (1 John 2:6 NET). Jesus said, "I have set you an example that you should do as I have done for you" (John 13:15). And Jesus, the only perfect, sinless person ever to live, practiced all but confession—which in His perfection He did not need.

If Jesus thought spiritual disciplines were critical for Himself, then we should strive to practice them ourselves—understanding that the gospel, for followers of Jesus, is built on not only disciplining ourselves for the purpose of godliness (1 Timothy 4:7) but also on the obedience of faith (Romans 1:5) and the fullness of joy (John 15:11).

20

DEVELOP AN ATTITUDE
OF GRATITUDE

One Thanksgiving, my wife, Barb, and I sat around the table after dinner with a small group of family and friends. One of our friends, who was away from her family, asked if we could practice a tradition her family had enjoyed for generations. "We go around in a circle," Ellen explained, "telling each other what we're thankful for. Each time you speak, you can only share one thing. We keep going around for as long as it takes."

I smiled but thought, *This probably won't take long.* Was I ever mistaken!

Ellen began. "Today I am grateful for a new family with which I can share this special holiday."

The next person in the circle continued. "Today I am grateful for a job I love."

"Today I am grateful for pumpkin pie and ice cream," said the next person. "Today I am grateful for a warm home," added another.

To my amazement, this simple exercise continued for more than 45 minutes, bringing much joy and laughter. As we cleared the table, you could hear individuals whistling or humming. Attitudes were positive—indeed, jolly.

We could have complained or gossiped or discussed our ills and problems; we could have concentrated on the difficult times our country has experienced—all of which would have depressed us. But Ellen demonstrated the principle that an attitude of gratitude almost always generates positive feelings and a sense of well-being.

Jayson D. Bradley writes, "The word 'gratitude' first showed up in the mid-fifteenth century. Adapted from the Latin word *gratitudinem*, which means 'thankfulness,' gratitude came to express deep, reciprocal appreciation for kindness received."[1] The ancient biblical narrative speaks abundantly about gratitude and being grateful (Jonah 2:9; Psalms 100; 118:28-29; 136:1-3; 147:7; Acts 24:3; Romans 6:4; Colossians 3:12-17; 1 Thessalonians 5:18). The words *thank(s)*, *thankful(ness)*, and *thanksgiving* appear in Scripture more than 170 times.

Writer G.K. Chesterton said, "When it comes to life, the critical thing is whether you take things for granted or take them with gratitude."[2] Frederic and Mary Ann Brussat wrote, "Gratitude puts everything in a fresh perspective; it enables us to see the many blessings all around us. And the more ways we give thanks, the more things we find to be grateful for. Giving thanks takes practice, however. We get better at it over time."[3]

I gave one of my patients who suffered from a particularly bad attitude (and the chronic depression that often goes with it) the assignment of keeping a daily gratitude journal for two weeks. Each evening she was to write down five things for which she was grateful or blessings she had experienced that day. On her next visit, she said, "I can't believe how much better it makes me feel and function. I still have bad moods and disappointments, but they seem to be getting better by the day. On days when I keep a list of all the little things that give me a lift, it's amazing how the good feelings just grow. On days when I forget… well, my bad attitude gets the best of me!"

Much research shows that an "attitude of gratitude" can immeasurably improve your overall well-being. Studies have shown that the positive benefits from simply giving heartfelt thanks can ease emotional burdens and stress, and that an attitude of gratitude helps people achieve high degrees of health and well-being (improved emotions), improved social behaviors and traits (improved relational health), and improvements in religiousness/spirituality (improved spiritual health).[4] There's a wonderful minute-and-a-half YouTube video from the

Templeton Foundation on the many health benefits of an attitude of gratitude as well as some tips on developing it at tinyurl.com/yal7fzdr.

When you find yourself brooding over an unpleasant experience, you can consciously choose to find a reason to be grateful or to consciously concentrate on a blessing in your life. By doing so, you perform your own therapy. The more you cultivate a positive coping style, the more likely you are to demonstrate feelings of well-being and happiness, no matter what your lot in life.

Here's our tip: keep a small journal at your bedside. For one week, each night before going to sleep, record five things for which you are grateful—the blessings you received that day. Then, for a minute or two, reflect on each item you recorded and thank God for the gifts you've been given. See what happens to your feelings. The next time something bad or irritating or disappointing happens to you—or the next time you find yourself brooding over an unpleasant experience—stop yourself. Choose instead—right away—to find a reason to be grateful. The Greater Good Science Center at UC Berkeley has a helpful article, "Tips for Keeping a Gratitude Journal," and will give you a digital gratitude journal at tinyurl.com/y7da7vo7.

Paul wrote,

> Rejoice in the Lord always. I will say it again: Rejoice! Let your gentleness be evident to all. The Lord is near. Do not be anxious about anything, but in every situation, by prayer and petition, with thanksgiving, present your requests to God. And the peace of God, which transcends all understanding, will guard your hearts and your minds in Christ Jesus. Brothers and sisters, whatever is true, whatever is noble, whatever is right, whatever is pure, whatever is lovely, whatever is admirable—if anything is excellent or praiseworthy—think about such things (Philippians 4:4-8).

Don't be surprised to find your attitude changes, you begin to develop a daily attitude of gratitude, and, as a result, you'll become more highly healthy!

21

READ MORE—
ESPECIALLY THE BIBLE

The editors of *Reader's Digest* write, "Here's a simple question—answer it honestly, because your response could boost the amount of pleasure in your daily life, delay dementia, and even help you live longer. How many hours did you spend reading last week?"[1]

They point out, "This question has arrived in thousands of American homes every other year since 1992 as part of the University of Michigan's Health and Retirement Study (HRS). A minor item on a massive survey of 20,000 retirees, it had been long ignored in the analysis of elder brain health."[2]

Then in 2016, Yale School of Public Health scientists dissected the HRS data about the "reading habits and health of more than 3,600 men and women over the age of 50." They discovered that "people who read books—fiction or nonfiction, poetry or prose—for as little as 30 minutes a day over several years were living an average of two years longer than people who didn't read anything at all."[3]

According to Huffpost.com, "Research conducted in 2009 at the University of Sussex showed reading was the most effective way to overcome stress, beating favorites such as listening to music, enjoying a cup of tea or coffee, and even taking a walk…Measured by evaluating heart rate and muscle tension, it took the study participants just six minutes to relax once they started turning pages."[4] In fact, after six minutes of reading, stress levels were reduced by 68 percent. Research shows that reading provides space for self-reflection,[5] increases levels of compassion,[6] and improves cognitive and overall health.[7]

Reading books, especially fiction, has been shown to increase empathy and emotional intelligence. Journalist Brandon Specktor writes, "One 2013 study found participants who read just the first part or chapter of a story showed a noticeable increase in empathy one week later, whereas news readers showed a decrease. These findings may sound trivial, but they're not; developing social tools such as empathy and emotional intelligence can lead to more (and more positive) human interaction, which in turn can lower stress levels—both of which are proved to help you live longer and healthier."[8]

He adds,

> Reading anything that fills your mind and exposes you to new words, phrases, and facts seems to carry mental benefits. New research indicates a large vocabulary may lead to a more resilient mind by fueling what scientists call *cognitive reserve*. We can think about this reserve as your brain's ability to adapt to damage. Cognitive reserve helps your brain cells find new mental pathways around areas damaged by stroke and dementia. This could explain why, after death, many seemingly healthy elders harbor advanced signs of Alzheimer's disease in their brains despite showing few signs in life. It's their cognitive reserve, researchers suspect, that may allow some seniors to compensate for hidden brain damage.[9]

So how does one build up cognitive reserve? Vocabulary has been shown to be highly resistant to aging, and having a rich vocabulary, according to researchers at the University of Santiago de Compostela, "can significantly delay the manifestation of mental decline. When the team analyzed vocabulary test scores of more than 300 volunteers ages 50 and older, they found participants with the lowest scores were between three and four times more at risk of cognitive decay than participants with the highest scores."[10]

Finding Good Reads

Most librarians love to help eager readers find good books. Your local library system is a good place to start. Pastors, church staff, friends, and family are also good sources. You can also join community and online book clubs.

In our view, an all-around great reading plan has to include the Bible. The Bible teaches us, "All Scripture is inspired by God and is useful for teaching, for showing people what is wrong in their lives, for correcting faults, and for teaching how to live right. Using the Scriptures, the person who serves God will be capable, having all that is needed to do every good work" (2 Timothy 3:16-17 NCV). Reading the Bible is good for you, and it will change you—for the better, forever. Jesus said, "It is written, 'Man shall not live by bread alone, but by every word that proceeds from the mouth of God'" (Matthew 4:4). He also says, "The words that I speak to you are spirit, and they are life" (John 6:63 NKJV).

God the Father, speaking of Jesus, told the disciples, "This is my Son, whom I love; with him I am well pleased. Listen to him!" (Matthew 17:5). We can find Jesus, listen to Jesus, and learn from Jesus no better way than by reading of His words and actions in the Gospels—as well as reading Scripture in general. Remember when Jesus, after His resurrection, was on the road to Emmaus with two disciples and "beginning with Moses and all the Prophets, he explained to them what was said in all the Scriptures concerning himself" (Luke 24:27).

Yet, of regular church attenders, only 45 percent read their Bible more than once a week, while more than 40 percent read their Bible occasionally, maybe once or twice a month, and almost one in five churchgoers say they never read the Bible at all.[11] Why is that?

The Institute for Bible Reading (IFBR) tells us, "Much of what makes up our modern Bible—chapters, verses, section heads, notes, commentary, cross-references, and red letters—has only been around for a few hundred years. The Bible used to be formatted like any other book. Now it looks more like an encyclopedia. Could the format influence how we read it?"[12]

In fact, research shows that the IFBR is correct because two habits make Bible reading less enjoyable and effective than it otherwise might be.[13]

1. Most read the Bible in tiny fragments rather than reading it book by book. Most read verse by verse or section by section or chapter by chapter—never finishing the author's thought.

2. Most read the Bible out of context. "Understanding the author's intended message for his original audience, understanding a book's place in the grand narrative of the Bible, and understanding the type of literature it is, are all critical to effective and enjoyable Bible reading." After all, the Bible admonishes each of us, "Do your best to present yourself to God as one approved, a worker who does not need to be ashamed and who correctly handles the word of truth" (2 Timothy 2:15).

The IFBR says, "We believe that the modern Bible format and unhealthy Bible reading practices are a big part of why so many people are struggling to read the Bible today."[14] No wonder more than half of American churchgoers admit to reading the Bible either occasionally or not at all.[15] What does IFBR suggest? They have created *Immerse: The Bible Reading Experience*, which is designed to help individuals and churches make regular, intentional Bible reading a core piece of their identity by using a Bible designed for reading at length.[16]

The IFBR says, "It starts with a new kind of Bible. Using all of the latest research on typography and page design, we created a Bible with one goal in mind: to provide the best reading experience possible. *Immerse: The Reading Bible* restores the Bible's text to its natural literary form: stories look like stories, songs look like songs, and poetry looks like poetry. Rather than traditional chapters and verses, each book is formatted based on the natural literary structures used when the books were first composed."[17]

In an article at WashingtonTimes.com, journalist Leland Ryken asks, "Why should we read the Bible as literature? Because its literary format requires it. C.S. Lewis…wrote in *Reflections on the Psalms* that 'there is a sense in which the Bible, since it is after all literature, cannot properly be read except as literature; and the different parts of it as the different sorts of literature they are.'"[18]

In some cases, the IFBR has reordered the books in a way that makes more sense for reading the Bible cover-to-cover as literature. This is what they say on their website, "We arranged the New Testament so that all four Gospels aren't bunched at the front, and Paul's letters are in approximate chronological order, rather than the traditional order of longest to shortest."[19]

IFBR recommends that small groups read sections of the Bible during the week and then get together to discuss what they've read. Scott Bolinder, the Executive Director of IFBR, writes:

> The communal aspect of *Immerse* seems to be an important part of deep engagement. Somehow, when we return to the ancient practice of "doing the Bible together in community," it allows the Holy Spirit to show up in organic ways and knit people together as they gather around the Text, and even wrestle together with the Text. Over and over, we hear about curiosity being renewed and imaginations rekindled as folks lose themselves in the Story. When people have read at length (dozens of pages a week), they are full and ready (yearning, even) to talk about what they've read with other kindred spirits.[20]

Barb and I have read an *Immerse* version, both in our private devotional time and with others in a small group. We loved it. You can learn more at tinyurl.com/yaah5kcy.

But the Bible is not just intended to be a good read. It is also designed to be God's handbook, manual, and guidebook for the path of our lives. Some use the acrostic BIBLE to remind them it can be God's Basic Instructions Before Leaving Earth. Receiving help from the Holy Spirit in understanding the Bible and learning to use the Bible to answer questions is a wise approach to becoming happier and healthier.

No one knows your situation like God, so who could be better equipped to answer all your questions? But you need to be able to find the right passages to fit your need and provide you guidance. K.W. Oliver's book *God's Handbook: Learn to Use the Bible to Answer All of Life's Most Difficult Questions!*[21] and Pastor Charles Stanley's book *Handbook for Christian Living: Biblical Answers to Life's Tough Questions*[22] are excellent resources to consider.

Nevertheless, as Jared C. Wilson points out, "We must never teach the practical points (of the Bible) as the main points. The practical stuff is always connected to the proclamational stuff. The 'dos' can never be detached from the 'done' of the finished work of Christ in the gospel, or else we run the risk of preaching the law." He adds, "Front to back, page to page, Genesis 1:1 to Revelation 22:21, the written Word of God is primarily and essentially about the saving revelation of the divine Word of God."[23]

For nearly five decades I've had the following quote in my Bible. It's attributed to Robert Chapman of Barnstable, Devonshire, England, who passed away at 99 years of age about 1903. I pray it will mean as much to you as it does me:[24]

> This Book contains the mind of God, the state of man, the way of salvation, doom of sinners, and happiness of believers.
>
> Its doctrines are holy, its precepts are binding, its histories are true, and its decisions are immutable.
>
> Read it to be wise, believe it to be safe, and practice it to be holy.
>
> It contains light to direct you, food to support you, and comfort to cheer you.
>
> It is the traveler's map, the pilgrim's staff, the pilot's compass, the soldier's sword, and the Christian's charter.
>
> Here paradise is restored, heaven opened, and the gates of hell disclosed.

Christ is its grand subject, our good its design, and the glory of God its end.

It should fill the memory, rule the heart, and guide the feet.

Read it slowly, frequently, prayerfully.

It is a mine of wealth, a paradise of glory, and a river of pleasure.

It is given you in life, will be open at the judgment, and be remembered forever.

It involves the highest responsibility, rewards the greatest labor, and condemns all who trifle with its holy contents.[25]

22

MEDITATE AND PRAY

n 2017 I wrote an article for health professionals titled "Praying with Our Patients," in which I said:

> For Christian healthcare professionals in particular, prayer is one of the most potent spiritual interventions we can utilize with our patients, not only because it has been shown by research to provide comfort for patients, but because we understand it is ultimately God who heals (Exodus 15:26).[1]

The Barna Group tells us, "Almost all American adults (94 percent) have prayed at least once in the last three months" and "most often choose to pray by themselves." They conclude, "Prayer is by far the most common spiritual practice among Americans."[2] And it's a highly healthy activity.

Harvard Medical School researcher Dr. Herbert Benson has both reviewed a plethora of studies and published others showing that the spiritual disciplines of prayer and meditation have multiple health benefits—showing, among other positive effects, that "people who meditate regularly enjoy lower stress levels, increased well-being, and even were able to reduce their blood pressure levels and resting heart rate."[3] Others have found a strong association between prayer and marital satisfaction and stability.[4] Still other researchers tell us that the health benefits of a quiet time, prayer, and meditation begin to accrue with an investment of as little as five to ten minutes a day.[5]

We believe it's likely that if you choose to invest more time, your health will improve even more. In essential 2, "Preventive Care," we suggest a simple formula for good health: 0-5-10-30-150. Can you remember what these numbers stand for? Zero cigarettes; five servings of fruit and vegetables a day; 10 minutes of silence, meditation, and prayer a day; a BMI of less than 30; and 150 minutes of exercise per week.[6] Prayer and meditation can affect all four wheels of your health.

Many medical studies have shown the significant effects of prayer and meditation. Studies show that prayer and meditation affect many health outcomes, including anxiety disorders, cardiovascular disease, depression, disabilities, marital satisfaction, pain relief, recovery from heart attack and surgery, intensive care unit stay duration, substance abuse, and generalized well-being. Studies have shown a positive correlation between activity such as prayer and satisfaction in life.[7]

One research group demonstrated the "strongest factors for well-being [life satisfaction and happiness] were frequency of prayer and prayer experience." They also found that conversational and meditative prayers were more strongly related to well-being than ritual or rote prayer.[8] Both talking with God (prayer) and listening to God (meditation and Bible reading) will increase your likelihood of becoming and remaining a happy, healthy person.

A study from the Pew Research Center found only about one-half of Americans pray daily[9]—and we would suggest that to pray infrequently is as unhealthy as breathing infrequently! In fact, Scripture tells us in 1 Thessalonians 5:17 to "pray continually" (NIV), or "pray without ceasing" (ESV), or "never stop praying" (NLT). US Senate Chaplain Barry C. Black writes, "The Greek word translated 'without ceasing' is *adialeiptos*, which doesn't mean nonstop—but actually means constantly recurring. In other words, we can punctuate our moments with intervals of recurring prayer."[10] He adds, "Ralph Waldo Emerson…in his sermon 'Pray Without Ceasing' made the following observation: 'Every secret wish is a prayer. Every house is a church; the corner of every street is a closet of devotion.'"[11]

It seems to us that too many Christians are overworked and underprayed!—meaning few of us "pray without ceasing." So even though we've discussed the value of prayer and meditation in essentials 2, 7, and 10, we want to reemphasize it here.

One of Phil's friends told him, "I am a person of action! But prayer... well, prayer is just so passive." He may think so but look at our Savior. Every time the disciples looked around, what did they see? Early in the morning, at midday, or in the evening, Immanuel, God-with-us, was praying. On another occasion, they were powerless to cure a sick little boy possessed by a demon. "After Jesus had gone indoors, His disciples asked Him privately, 'Why couldn't we drive it out?' He replied, 'This kind can come out only by prayer'" (Mark 9:28-29).

Why are we powerless? Many Christians take prayer lightly and pray infrequently—perhaps just saying grace over meals. The late Howard Hendricks used to say, "Invite a magician to church and you will pack the place. Call a prayer meeting, and people will stay away in droves!"[12]

Jesus's disciples finally caught on to the power of prayer and asked Jesus, "Lord, teach us to pray, just as John taught his disciples" (Luke 11:1). Prayer...passive? We don't think so! Paul exhorts us, "Pray in the Spirit on all occasions with all kinds of prayers and requests. With this in mind, be alert and always keep on praying for all the Lord's people" (Ephesians 6:18-19).

Jesus, who is God the Son in the flesh, was consistently talking and listening to the Father. Yet we, who don't know much about the God who created us, are too busy to pray! It has been said, "If you are too busy to pray, you are too busy!"[13]

And what about this meditation stuff? Well, meditation is simply taking the time to think about what we know and are learning about God. God speaks in and through Scripture, and it may take a little while to wrap our minds around what the God of the universe is communicating to us.

How to Pray and Meditate

Crosswalk.com contributor Kelly O'Dell Stanley says, "Here's the good news. Not only is it possible to pray without ceasing, but it's possible to do so without making any significant changes to your schedule or time commitments. It's all about shifting your thought process and turning everyday moments into prayer." She suggests nine ways to pray without ceasing:[14]

1. *Begin with gratitude.* Start by telling God what you're thankful for. Prayer doesn't have to be asking for something. It can simply be thanking Him from your heart for what He has already done.

2. *Get real.* Prayer is simply a conversation. Talk to Him the way you would talk to a friend. Let the words pour out casually and simply. Just be real.

3. *Incorporate prayer into everyday chores.* Let your everyday tasks become acts of worship by turning them into times of prayer.

4. *Tell Him what He already knows.* God already knows what's in our hearts, but when we offer our thoughts to Him, it turns what might be a solitary life into a richer, more meaningful relationship. And I think God delights in this.

5. *Pray while you wait.* Most of us waste a lot of time while we wait. A quick online search reports that we each average two years of our lives waiting in line, and the average commuter spends 38 hours a year in traffic. Turn your wait times and car commute into a prayer closet. Transform that time into something meaningful. Pray for the people you expect to encounter that day or the tasks you need to accomplish. Pray especially for those drivers who cut you off or fail to signal a turn. Give thanks, count your blessings—because they're everywhere—and make those minutes count.

6. *Sing songs of praise.* "Is anyone among you in trouble? Let them pray. Is anyone happy? Let them sing songs of praise" (James 5:13). Remember the idea of prayer being like a radio playing in the background all the time. Make that literal by listening to worship music. As you sing along, offer the words to God as your prayer.

7. *When you mess up, admit it.* We don't know about you, but we could spend most of our praying-without-ceasing time simply confessing a litany of our sins and failings. When we confess, God forgives us, so we don't need to dwell there. (That in itself is another reason to praise Him.)

8. *Give up worrying.* Philippians 4:6 says, "Do not be anxious about anything, but in every situation, by prayer and petition, with thanksgiving, present your requests to God." We're not meant to worry, and we waste too many minutes doing just that. Next time something weighs heavy on your heart, envision yourself extending it up to God and letting Him hold it for you. Ask Him what your role is and if there is something you need to do. If so, do it. But don't take back the weight of the worry. Then start thanking God for who He is and what He has already done for you, and you'll feel the weight lifting off your shoulders as the words come.

9. *Stop talking once in a while.* Instead, just listen. Spend some of your praying-without-ceasing time just being— simply sitting and resting in His presence. Keep in mind that the best conversations are two-sided, but you won't hear anything if you never stop to listen.

James wrote, "My dear brothers and sisters, take note of this: Everyone should be quick to listen, slow to speak" (James 1:19). A frequent quote on the internet (for which we have not found a source) is: "Worry is conversation you have with yourself about things you cannot change; prayer is a conversation you have with God about things He can change." One cannot worry and trust God at the same time.

Prayer and meditation demand two elements described in a plaque at the Ignatius House, a Jesuit retreat center in Atlanta that hosts silent retreats: "LISTEN & SILENT have the same letters. Coincidence?"[15] We suggest beginning prayer and meditation with what Matthew Henry called *The Prayer of Samuel:*[16] "Speak, for your servant is listening"

(1 Samuel 3:10). You can ask your Father in heaven to speak to you through His Word (Hebrews 4:12), His creation (Psalm 19:1-4), your circumstances (Colossians 4:3; Revelation 3:8), other people (Acts 2:14-41), and His Spirit (Acts 16:6-10).

Besides praying without ceasing, we recommend you schedule your own personal, private times to pray—just as Jesus did. Mark recorded, "Very early in the morning, while it was still dark, Jesus got up, left the house and went off to a solitary place, where he prayed" (Mark 1:35). If you don't put it in your schedule, it won't get done. If you are new to prayer, listen to experienced prayers. Read the prayers of Jesus and others in Scripture. Read the prayers of godly men and women who have recorded those for us. Speak to God—but also be careful to listen to Him.

We also recommend you seek out scheduled opportunities to pray with other Christians on a regular basis. Sometimes finding such a group may be a bit of a challenge, but it will be worth it.

Meditation does not mean *emptying* the mind, but rather filling it with God's thoughts and God's Word. It requires substance to meditate upon. If you are reading Scripture, listening to sermons, and participating in Bible studies, Sunday school, and small groups, your aim in all these activities is to hear from God. When you hear, you need to think about what you are hearing. Ask yourself questions such as:

- How does this impact/apply to me?
- How do I apply this truth in my life?
- What does this truth tell me about God? About my fellow man?
- What do I need to change immediately?
- What message does the God of the universe have for me personally?

Paul reminds each of us, "Do not conform to the pattern of this world but be transformed by the renewing of your mind" (Romans 12:2). Praying, meditating upon, and memorizing God's Word can do just that.

I have cared for thousands of patients in my 40 years of medical practice. One thing I've noticed in my older Christian patients is that as they grow more physically and mentally frail, they come to realize that they have more interest in developing the ministry of praying, meditating, and practicing the presence of God. Instead of fading away, they become prayer warriors for the Lord.

In Colossians 4:2, Paul writes: "Devote yourselves to prayer, being watchful and thankful." Jesus told us we "should always pray and not give up" (Luke 18:1), and God, the Father, speaking of Jesus told the apostles, "This is my Son, whom I love. Listen to him!" (Mark 9:7). We each should consider imitating Him in prayer and listening to Him and His Word in meditation.

To sum up, our prayer for you and your loved ones is that you would become fit over 50 by making everyday choices from our medically reliable and biblically sound 10 essentials and 22 tips to become a happier (more blessed) and healthier you. We finish by joining the apostle John in this prayer for you: "Dear friend, I pray that you may enjoy good health and that all may go well with you, even as your soul is getting along well" (3 John 1:2).

Acknowledgments

An amazing group of health professionals critically reviewed the manuscript to help us assure you it was up to date, trustworthy, and medically reliable. We are grateful to:

Cardiology: Steven Brown, MD, PhD, FACC and Daniel Van-Hamersveld, MD, FACC

Dermatology: Robert D Griffith, MD, FAAD

Emergency Medicine: Adrian Blackwell, MD, DABEM and Michael Bishop, MD, FACEP

Exercise Science and Sports Performance: Alicia T. Bryan, PhD, FACSM (Kinesiology) and Tim Dornemann EdD, CES, PES, CSCS

Family Medicine: Jennifer K. Allen, MD, DABFM; Marc A. Chetta, MD, FAAFP; James D. Collier, MD; Susan Henriksen, MD; Keith Horwood, MD, DABFM; Julian Hsu, MD, FAAFP; Chris Jenkins, MD; Sarah S. Jones, MD, FAAFP; Thomas A. Kintinar, MD, FAAFP; Patricia Landry, MD; Edward Langston, MD, FAAFP (Former Chair, Board of Trustees, American Medical Association); Huy Q. Luu, DO, DABFM; Thomas L. McKnight, MD; Dale E. Michaels, MD, DABFM; M. Shawn Morehead, MD, FAAFP; Cherec Morrison, MD; John A. Mulder, MD, FAAHPM, HMDC; Mary Anne Nelson, MD, FAAFP; Daniel J. Ostergaard, MD, FAAFP; Robert Low Ridley, MD; Edward E. Rylander, MD, DABFM, DABHPM; Cathie Scarbrough, MD, FAAFP; Chuck Schoephoerster, PAC; Roshini Isabell Selladurai, MD; and Robert Vogt, MD, DABFM

Gastroenterology: Erik Van Os, MD

Internal Medicine/Pediatrics: David Kim, MD and Janet Kim, MD, MA (bioethics)

Mental health: Dwight Bain, LMHC, NCC, CPC; Bill Maier, PsyD; Barbara Seeds, MA (psychology), MFT; and Juli Slattery, PhD

Nutrition and Dietetics: Cheryl Flynt, RD, LDN (Manager, Center for Nutritional Excellence, Florida Hospital, Orlando, FL); and Kelly Pritchett PhD, RDN, CSSD (Board Certified Specialist in Sports Nutrition)

Obstetrics and Gynecology: Fred Brown, MD, FACOG; and Steve Foley, MD, FACOG

Pediatrics: Janet Kim, MD

Psychiatry: Karl Benzio, MD, DABPN and Marisa Giggie, MD, MPA (General, Child, & Adolescent, and Forensic Psychiatry)

Public health: Reginald Finger, MD, MPH; Cheryl Flynt, RD, LDN, MPH; Marisa Giggie, MD, MPA; Dilip Joseph, MD, MPH; David Kim, MD, MBA (healthcare); Janet Kim, MD, MPH; Thomas L. McKnight, MD, MPH; M. Shawn Morehead, MD, MPH; Mike Perko, PhD; Chuck Schoephoerster, MPH, PAC; and Eric Walsh, MD, DrPH

Pulmonology and Critical Care Medicine: Peter Hountras, MD, FACP, FCCP

Radiology: Susan M. Griffith, MD, ACR, ABNM

Surgery: Michael Chupp, MD, FACS, FCS (ECSA, General Surgery, CEO, Christian Medical and Dental Associations); Daniel Henriksen, MD, FACS; Sally Knox, MD, FACS; and Barry D. Newsom, MD, FACS (Thoracic and Cardiovascular Surgery)

Biblical Interpretation and Theology: Teaching Pastor David Erickson, MA, MMin; Chris Jenkins, MD, MDiv, ThM; Thomas L. McKnight, MDiv; Senior Pastor Buz McNutt, PhD; Danny Loe, ThM, DMin; Senior Pastor Bryan Myers, MMin; Senior Pastor Jon Quitt; Senior Pastor Chris Taylor, EdS, MAMFC, MARE; and Stan W. Wallace, DMin

I heard Michael Card say early in his career that he had never published lyrics or a book not reviewed and approved by his home church's elder board. I was so impressed by that accountability that I've had every one of my 30 plus books reviewed the same way. So I'm grateful to the elder board of my home church, Academy Christian Church in Colorado Springs, Colorado (Pastors Bryan Myers and Dave Erickson, Craig Butterfield, David F. Smith, Jim Collier, Larry Jacob, Larry Lawrence, Mike Folkerts, Richard Crabtree, and Steve McFarland), for their review and counsel. Thanks also to Don Jones of Studio 9 Commercial Photography for allowing me to use a portrait he took of me. You can see his amazing work at tinyurl.com/y3nkdkku.

Thanks to our agent, Greg Johnson, founder and president of WordServe Literary, who worked so diligently to find a home for this book. We are blessed by God to have this opportunity to work with Harvest House to make this information available to you. A special thanks to our talented senior acquisitions editor, Todd Hafer. Senior editor Kim Moore was the project manager and an amazing encourager and cheerleader (Thanks, Kim!), and Jennifer McNeil was our eagle-eyed line editor (and did she ever make the book better!). Any remaining mistakes are completely ours! Our appreciation goes also to Kari Galloway, who oversaw the design process, and Heather Green, Michael Bennet, Adrienne Hedlund, and Jeff Marion of our marketing team.

We especially appreciate the support of our families and most especially our wives, Barb Larimore and Brenda Bishop, for their support, prayers, and endless edits. We appreciate, most of all, the Lord Jesus Christ, who delivered us from the domain of darkness and transferred us to His kingdom (Colossians 1:13).

Walt Larimore
Phil Bishop

BIBLE PERMISSIONS

NOTES

PART ONE—10 Essentials

1. Balance

1. Walt Larimore, *10 Essentials of Happy, Healthy People* (Grand Rapids, MI: Zondervan, 2003).
2. Ibid. 34-36.
3. tinyurl.com/y998lald
4. tinyurl.com/ybgklfjt
5. Quoted from: tinyurl.com/y9snju4a
6. Ibid.
7. tinyurl.com/ycjkhe54
8. tinyurl.com/y7tntsc3
9. tinyurl.com/y9drcdz7
10. tinyurl.com/y9snju4a
11. tinyurl.com/yaoq7klv
12. Ibid.
13. tinyurl.com/y88wztaq
14. tinyurl.com/auqchza
15. tinyurl.com/bejyhq3

2. Preventive Care

1. tinyurl.com/y72duvox
2. tinyurl.com/hyr2kok
3. tinyurl.com/ybt5mmfj
4. tinyurl.com/y97yjr7t
5. Quoted from: tinyurl.com/y9vjund6
6. Adapted from: tinyurl.com/y2tuoh9z
7. tinyurl.com/ycfsmoc2
8. tinyurl.com/y9levvs5
9. tinyurl.com/hscqdv8
10. tinyurl.com/y7l3abwf
11. tinyurl.com/y27rn89l
12. tinyurl.com/y99xr5ls
13. tinyurl.com/yx9e4kyh
14. tinyurl.com/hscqdv8
15. tinyurl.com/ycm2xfh7
16. tinyurl.com/ybsaoyo9

17. tinyurl.com/yczhp28p
18. tinyurl.com/ybsaoyo9
19. tinyurl.com/ybw7e9u4
20. tinyurl.com/y72duvox
21. tinyurl.com/y6weu2on
22. Ibid.
23. tinyurl.com/y2gstpja
24. tinyurl.com/ycbwudn2
25. Quoted from: tinyurl.com/y7ur48bc
26. Adapted from: tinyurl.com/y72duvox
27. tinyurl.com/y84tbgwf
28. Adapted from: Ibid. See also tinyurl.com/y56lm4v8
29. tinyurl.com/y7qetlhp
30. tinyurl.com/ycgpdsrz

3. Forgiveness

1. tinyurl.com/y8n27tp5
2. tinyurl.com/y8hx6b7z
3. tinyurl.com/y8n27tp5
4. tinyurl.com/y9c9y47h
5. tinyurl.com/y8n27tp5
6. Ibid.
7. tinyurl.com/yargta52
8. tinyurl.com/y72h6tfn
9. tinyurl.com/yczcvw3n
10. tinyurl.com/yamse9sk
11. tinyurl.com/yc5ytc6z
12. tinyurl.com/y3l2xkul
13. tinyurl.com/yd6gvr7n
14. tinyurl.com/yc5ytc6z
15. Danny Loe, personal communication, October 24, 2018.
16. tinyurl.com/y92s5n6q
17. tinyurl.com/yargta52
18. tinyurl.com/y7ffp9d7

19. tinyurl.com/yazbx3ju
20. tinyurl.com/ycf7vqq6
21. tinyurl.com/y9varvhu
22. tinyurl.com/y76jz2dq

4. Reduce S-A-D-ness

1. Walt Larimore, *10 Essentials of Happy, Healthy People* (Grand Rapids, MI: Zondervan, 2003), 111-4.
2. tinyurl.com/y7bpd77l
3. tinyurl.com/ycj7u3tn
4. tinyurl.com/yaovzzvn
5. tinyurl.com/px8yl4m
6. tinyurl.com/y5qqqaem, tinyurl.com/y5fjp89g
7. tinyurl.com/yc4sqocd
8. tinyurl.com/yc4hszzq
9. tinyurl.com/y7jgsclk
10. tinyurl.com/ydx8ed4n
11. Reverend Rodney Wood, "The Letter I Began Writing on the First Day of my 69th Year," personal communication, September 28, 2018.
12. Barbara Seeds, personal communication, October 16, 2018.
13. tinyurl.com/y9ma4fof
14. tinyurl.com/y78vqjgo
15. tinyurl.com/ycgg65z6
16. tinyurl.com/yblp22qc
17. tinyurl.com/y4he6pgf
18. tinyurl.com/y78vqjgo
19. tinyurl.com/ycubn5xq
20. tinyurl.com/y9vu4x54
21. tinyurl.com/ybks5yz8
22. tinyurl.com/y9luewf2
23. tinyurl.com/ybnaqffn
24. tinyurl.com/ydd7kfrs
25. tinyurl.com/zuzvmme
26. tinyurl.com/ybda2jaq
27. tinyurl.com/y75r8gdb
28. tinyurl.com/ydyfts32
29. Ibid.
30. tinyurl.com/y9xykvv7

31. tinyurl.com/ybo9qbhy
32. tinyurl.com/y9qj3x73
33. tinyurl.com/yxpeto6
34. tinyurl.com/ybxwjz83
35. tinyurl.com/yckx7w6e
36. tinyurl.com/yatf3dd8
37. Adapted from: tinyurl.com/y3fbru38
38. tinyurl.com/y8c4wyr7

5. Healthy Relationships

1. tinyurl.com/yxeedv6j
2. tinyurl.com/yd8dnjkf
3. tinyurl.com/yaydwpxu
4. tinyurl.com/y4magwb2
5. Ibid.
6. tinyurl.com/y89uhcon
7. tinyurl.com/y6ue3pv6
8. tinyurl.com/yaugw3d3
9. Joe Battaglia, *Unfriended: Finding True Community in a Disconnected Culture* (New York, NY: Broadstreet, 2018), 122.
10. Battaglia, *Unfriended,* back cover liner.
11. tinyurl.com/yb9lztoj
12. Ibid.
13. tinyurl.com/yc3rhewq
14. tinyurl.com/nyr7gak
15. tinyurl.com/ybhych76
16. tinyurl.com/hfw6cu7
17. tinyurl.com/ybtnyv3y
18. tinyurl.com/ycqva398
19. tinyurl.com/ybtnyv3y
20. tinyurl.com/yabz9gbg
21. tinyurl.com/yaszucds
22. tinyurl.com/yc4el9f8
23. tinyurl.com/y6vbtbrx
24. tinyurl.com/y5n4fj5q
25. tinyurl.com/ybpdjzw5
26. tinyurl.com/y3fbru38
27. tinyurl.com/ybhych76
28. tinyurl.com/ybosldyh
29. Dr. Reginald Finger, personal communication, October 16, 2018.

30. tinyurl.com/y89uhcon

31. Barna Group, "Most People Seek Control, Adventure, and Peace in Their Lives," *Barna Updates*, (August 1, 2000).

32. tinyurl.com/ybtxuaob

33. tinyurl.com/y8gdw2f5

34. tinyurl.com/y8gdw2f5

6. Spiritual Well-Being

1. tinyurl.com/yc8q8zor

2. John K. Ryan, trans., *The Confessions of St. Augustine* (New York, NY: Image Books Doubleday, 2018), 43.

3. Bishop Edmond Lee Browning, *A Year of Days with the Book of Common Prayer* (New York, NY: Ballantine, 1997).

4. tinyurl.com/y7v4cjqx

5. tinyurl.com/y7v4cjqx

6. tinyurl.com/y7tlw343

7. tinyurl.com/y7s2evdk

8. Dale Matthews and Connie Clark, *The Faith Factor: Proof of the Healing Power of Prayer* (New York, NY: Viking, 1998), 54.

9. tinyurl.com/ycqy2jpu

10. Barna Updates, "People's Faith Flavor Influences How They See Themselves" (August 26, 2002).

11. Barna, "People's Faith Flavor Influences How They See Themselves."

12. tinyurl.com/y7tntsc3

13. tinyurl.com/y6wxbawo

14. tinyurl.com/yb2zjey2: pages 217-18

7. Positive Self-Image

1. tinyurl.com/yd5w575w

2. tinyurl.com/yaw2tffs

3. tinyurl.com/y8pgdglx

4. tinyurl.com/ycsa6fsw

5. tinyurl.com/y2fj5kv5

6. tinyurl.com/y5evevw2

7. tinyurl.com/y8f5popl

8. tinyurl.com/zfw6aoz

9. John Piper, *Don't Waste Your Life* (Wheaton, IL: Crossway, 2003), 33-34.

10. tinyurl.com/y42srxme

11. tinyurl.com/yy58ehf5

12. tinyurl.com/yyrxzmaj

13. tinyurl.com/yxs7y63k

14. tinyurl.com/y2e4jfwb

15. Harold G. Koenig, Dana E. King, and Verna B. Carson, *Handbook of Religion and Health* 2nd ed. (New York: Oxford University Press, 2012): 125, 151, 160, 163, 166, 173, 332, 355, 366, 368.

16. tinyurl.com/yy58ehf5

17. tinyurl.com/ycl8qdm5

18. tinyurl.com/y43rruoe

19. Steve Wilson, "Happiness Is an Inside Job," quoted in Walt Larimore, *10 Essentials of Happy, Healthy People* (Grand Rapids, MI: Zondervan, 2003), 290.

20. tinyurl.com/y3umxb3s

21. Thomas L. McKnight, personal communication, October 23, 2018.

22. Henri J. M. Nouwen, *Spiritual Direction: Wisdom for the Long Walk of Faith* (New York, NY: HarperCollins, 2006), 32-33.

23. tinyurl.com/y2pd5odf

24. tinyurl.com/yb9q6cq5

25. tinyurl.com/y3f5xxph

26. tinyurl.com/y6hxoz4s

27. tinyurl.com/y29ldwkw

8. Uncover Your Passion

1. Frank Minirth, Paul Meier, Richard Meier, and Don Hawkins, *The Healthy Christian Life* (Grand Rapids, MI: Baker, 1988), 25-26.

2. Richard Leider, *The Power of Purpose: Creating Meaning in Your Life and Work* (San Francisco, CA: Berrett-Koehler, 1997), 30.

3. Kurt Bruner, *The Divine Drama* (Wheaton, IL: Tyndale House, 2002).

4. Bill and Kathy Peel, *Discover Your Destiny: Finding the Courage to Follow Your Dreams* (Colorado Springs, CO: NavPress, 1997).

5. tinyurl.com/y9kma9jz

6. Patricia Landry, personal communication, October 23, 2018.

7. Thomas Edison, quoted in Héctor Amézquita, *Unleashing Thought Power and the Power of Believing* (Victoria, Canada: Trafford Publishing, 2003), 119.

8. tinyurl.com/y8axfbcj

9. B.J. Slomoff, "Embrace life: Fulfill your life purpose," *Hawaii Dental Journal* 32, no. 4 (2001): 9.

9. Personal Responsibility

1. Ibid.

2. Walt Larimore, *10 Essentials of Highly Healthy People* (Grand Rapids, MI: Zondervan, 2003), 223-8.

3. Joel E. Yeager, MD, *Transforming Healthcare Together: A Model for Restoring the Covenant of Trust* (Pennsauken, NJ: BookBaby, 2018).

4. tinyurl.com/yyrfvrk8

5. tinyurl.com/y3wa5ggf

6. Order of St. Luke (tinyurl.com/y9t5bvcq). The International Order of St. Luke the Physician is a Christian healing ministry and fellowship of (1) professional people in all phases of medical work; (2) clergy in the ministry of the Roman, Orthodox, Anglican, and Protestant churches; and (3) laypeople from all walks of life who believe that the healing ministry of Jesus Christ belongs in the church today. The order is the outgrowth of the Fellowship of Saint Luke, begun in 1932 by the late John Gayner Banks, S.T.D., priest of the Episcopal Church, and his wife, Ethel Tulloch Banks.

7. Stephen Ministry (tinyurl.com/cg6djuq). For more than 25 years, Stephen Ministries has been serving thousands of congregations from more than one hundred denominations with biblical, Christ-centered training and resources for one-to-one lay care giving, small groups, and spiritual growth and healing.

10. Your Healthcare Team

1. tinyurl.com/y9t62thf

2. tinyurl.com/ycklwj9q

3. Dónal O'Mathúna and Walt Larimore. *Alternative Medicine: The Christian Handbook. Updated and Expanded* (Grand Rapids, MI: Zondervan, 2006).

4. tinyurl.com/y2m74p5w

5. tinyurl.com/y6weu2on

6. tinyurl.com/y6yocz8s, tinyurl.com/y4nmplyy, tinyurl.com/y7n6fwea

7. tinyurl.com/y7n6fwea

8. Paul Meier, *Don't Let Jerks Get the Best of You: Advice for Dealing with Difficult People* (Nashville, TN: Thomas Nelson, 1995).

9. Jan Silvious, *Fool-Proofing Your Life: Wisdom for Untangling Your Most Difficult Relationships* (Colorado Springs, CO: WaterBrook, 1998).

PART TWO—
22 Tips for a Happier, Healthier You

RELATIONAL HEALTH TIPS

1. Tend to Others: Love Your Neighbor

1. tinyurl.com/yayek3m5

2. tinyurl.com/y5ncb3hq

3. tinyurl.com/yxlo4x5b

2. Volunteer—for Your Health

1. tinyurl.com/y8cx9opt

2. tinyurl.com/ycl56c2h

3. tinyurl.com/jhs62v4

4. tinyurl.com/y7m7oay4

5. tinyurl.com/yxk34aaz

6. tinyurl.com/h4o8zwc

7. tinyurl.com/yd5syncy

3. Get a Workout Buddy or Buddies

1. tinyurl.com/y7zbsnw4

2. Ibid.

4. Rediscover Sex—with Your Spouse

1. tinyurl.com/y9txo2nk

2. Ibid.

3. tinyurl.com/y76l6yr7

4. tinyurl.com/ydcel5vb

5. tinyurl.com/y8kh7v3l

6. tinyurl.com/y7y4g4oj

7. Quoted from: tinyurl.com/yb7lo6k6

8. Ibid.

9. Adapted from: tinyurl.com/y8kh7v3l

10. tinyurl.com/j4d4xvx

11. tinyurl.com/y7x6ulh2

12. tinyurl.com/y9hobp8t

13. tinyurl.com/y87j36jt

14. tinyurl.com/y5x86kz8

15. tinyurl.com/y87j36jt

16. tinyurl.com/yb7lo6k6

17. tinyurl.com/y6uaf3qh

18. tinyurl.com/yblb5bjt

EMOTIONAL HEALTH TIPS

5. Get a Pet—or Two!

1. tinyurl.com/yccw2we3

2. tinyurl.com/o9ns6dz

3. Adapted from: tinyurl.com/y8e3vbxx

4. tinyurl.com/y8vlgo3x

5. tinyurl.com/ydy2k2u7

6. tinyurl.com/yccw2we3

7. tinyurl.com/y94natq6

8. tinyurl.com/ycmaesnu

9. tinyurl.com/yccw2we3

10. Ibid.

11. tinyurl.com/y7kj2cye

12. tinyurl.com/yajujgcy

13. tinyurl.com/yd2rwp26

14. tinyurl.com/y8wy9j42

15. tinyurl.com/yarm58zt

16. Quoted from: tinyurl.com/ydektc5e

17. tinyurl.com/yarm58zt

18. tinyurl.com/y7vdbzm5

6. Get Outdoors

1. tinyurl.com/ycj2m52t

2. tinyurl.com/yavnejp5

3. tinyurl.com/ybazmv5z

4. tinyurl.com/y5wepg7u

5. tinyurl.com/ybazmv5z

6. Ibid.

7. Ibid.

8. tinyurl.com/nwz8xjl

9. Ibid.

10. tinyurl.com/y6anf8q9

11. tinyurl.com/ybnkakm9

12. tinyurl.com/y3dp4cua

13. tinyurl.com/ybrd7vh9

14. tinyurl.com/y4hpa35y

15. tinyurl.com/y7xelb6w

16. tinyurl.com/yd2ybr6v

17. Ibid.

18. tinyurl.com/ydxk9woh

19. tinyurl.com/yxvqwzh5

7. Get Your Mind in Shape

1. tinyurl.com/yyxflnar

2. Adapted from: tinyurl.com/y7782u8d

3. tinyurl.com/ya742yxb

4. tinyurl.com/y6w7zvyc

5. tinyurl.com/y839o9ou

6. tinyurl.com/yccv4jmn

7. tinyurl.com/yasc9u7b

8. tinyurl.com/y8s5n5r3

9. tinyurl.com/y49zj3dv

10. tinyurl.com/y5suyvld

11. tinyurl.com/ya7erz9u

12. tinyurl.com/ybpwscq5

13. tinyurl.com/yawdj9fl

14. tinyurl.com/yc8pmqgq

15. tinyurl.com/yawdj9fl

16. Quote from and list adapted from: tinyurl.com/yan4squz

17. tinyurl.com/yan4squz

18. tinyurl.com/y9ma4fof

19. tinyurl.com/y7782u8d

20. Kitty Crenshaw and Cathy Snapp, PhD, *The Hidden Life Awakened* (Jacksonville, FL: Cairnes Resources, 2016), xiii.

8. Enjoy the Rewards of Aging

1. tinyurl.com/y9j8c6yk

2. tinyurl.com/y9db72c5

3. tinyurl.com/yaryt9te

4. Ibid.

5. tinyurl.com/ybkduy39

6. tinyurl.com/yyxkr755

7. tinyurl.com/ybselu5a

8. tinyurl.com/ycftv7k9

9. tinyurl.com/y2eymd85

10. Ibid.

11. tinyurl.com/y4j8rwgn

12. tinyurl.com/kty6sqo

PHYSICAL HEALTH TIPS

9. Five Habits to Live Ten Years Longer (or More)!

1. tinyurl.com/pak4ca8

2. tinyurl.com/y89yuj3t

3. Adapted from: Ibid.

4. tinyurl.com/yac3bd3v

5. tinyurl.com/y8xnzr9u

6. tinyurl.com/y55y5qrs

7. tinyurl.com/y7t6zmf2

8. tinyurl.com/y8xnzr9u].

9. tinyurl.com/y9o2yvdh

10. tinyurl.com/y7fvv94q

11. tinyurl.com/y8epmd5w

12. tinyurl.com/ydgssgug

10. You Need to Know Four Numbers

1. tinyurl.com/yby2qvqa

2. tinyurl.com/ycqeh6kc

3. Ibid.

4. tinyurl.com/y9xvmb9d

5. tinyurl.com/z5rapdl

6. tinyurl.com/y84tbgwf

7. tinyurl.com/y8qd9qj6

8. tinyurl.com/y9hokww5

9. tinyurl.com/yc6lkm6k

10. tinyurl.com/y9hokww5

11. tinyurl.com/yc6lkm6k

12. tinyurl.com/y9hokww5

13. tinyurl.com/yc6lkm6k

14. tinyurl.com/y9hokww5

15. tinyurl.com/y9vjund6

16. Quoted from: tinyurl.com/y9zwcunf

11. Eat like a Greek

1. tinyurl.com/ycbpyo3r

2. tinyurl.com/yb8uzb94

3. tinyurl.com/y29uo8vp

4. tinyurl.com/yd53cmg4

5. tinyurl.com/ybsmjqzv

6. tinyurl.com/ycbpyo3r

7. tinyurl.com/yb9wcqb6

8. tinyurl.com/ybybkphm

9. tinyurl.com/yc6nbarz

10. tinyurl.com/ycfrux8b

11. tinyurl.com/y3ryjx4b

12. tinyurl.com/y6lohchx

12. Move!

1. tinyurl.com/y7czfja6
2. tinyurl.com/y8e6jdfx
3. tinyurl.com/y8ghau37
4. tinyurl.com/ybsw9yga
5. tinyurl.com/yacghg4x
6. tinyurl.com/yb2zopzp
7. tinyurl.com/y8z2n6gz
8. tinyurl.com/y7so7jhl
9. Ibid.
10. tinyurl.com/ybz7pf87
11. tinyurl.com/y7j67xkx
12. tinyurl.com/yc29mxqs
13. tinyurl.com/ybvnonoj
14. tinyurl.com/y9qnlzh9
15. Ibid.
16. tinyurl.com/y9qeqmm4
17. tinyurl.com/ybfohted
18. tinyurl.com/y7z4o29r
19. tinyurl.com/y8o4t6e6
20. Quoted from: tinyurl.com/y7pauzb6
21. tinyurl.com/yawuvv7u
22. tinyurl.com/yb3wuehx
23. tinyurl.com/yd65dbrw
24. tinyurl.com/ydx34gjk
25. tinyurl.com/y8nxmy76
26. tinyurl.com/y8syh4tk
27. tinyurl.com/y79b2l6j
28. tinyurl.com/ydgjdy67
29. tinyurl.com/y8tstuzt
30. tinyurl.com/y9mxnl5r
31. tinyurl.com/y3ze2ujb
32. tinyurl.com/yatg7trl
33. Connie Jankowski, *Hippocrates: Father of Medicine* (North Mankato, MN: Compass Point Books, 2009), 24.
34. Adapted from: tinyurl.com/y7de8hny
35. Ibid.
36. Adapted from: tinyurl.com/y8z2xqq3
37. tinyurl.com/yb5uxcnq
38. tinyurl.com/y6pmxoxk
39. tinyurl.com/yyt4gsfk
40. tinyurl.y6xhnbvp
41. tinyurl.com/y3xukkqu
42. Ibid.
43. tinyurl.com/ya5dmdjp
44. tinyurl.com/yazwsr8x
45. tinyurl.com/y7qfa2qb
46. tinyurl.com/yayc8het
47. tinyurl.com/y2h5u47x
48. Bradford Torrey, ed., *The Writings of Henry David Thoreau: 1837–1946* (New York: Houghton Mifflin and Company), chapter VII (1845–1846), 134.

13. Flexibility—More Important Than Ever

1. tinyurl.com/yd289yvj
2. tinyurl.com/yycvn5cd
3. tinyurl.com/yd6xz8n7
4. tinyurl.com/ya6gwzpw

14. Lifting Weights Is Not Just for Athletes

1. Adapted from: tinyurl.com/yazprw2y
2. tinyurl.com/ybbdbjpp
3. tinyurl.com/y9ohj3g3
4. tinyurl.com/y8kfsp5a
5. tinyurl.com/ybs6l89x

15. Tips to Avoid Colorectal Cancer

1. tinyurl.com/y83hyo46
2. tinyurl.com/y8vst4mp
3. Ibid.
4. tinyurl.com/y7q53ulv
5. tinyurl.com/ya3kuce2
6. tinyurl.com/y7ufqzcf
7. tinyurl.com/y8vst4mp
8. Ibid.
9. Ibid.
10. tinyurl.com/yaazpp5u
11. "Natural Medicines in the Clinical Management of Colon Cancer," Clinical Management Series, NMCD Website, subscription required), tinyurl.com/ycj6lcsv
12. tinyurl.com/y8vst4mp
13. tinyurl.com/ya7o2qrb

14. tinyurl.com/y98krq3u
15. tinyurl.com/y7tmjw7n
16. tinyurl.com/y8msyz68
17. tinyurl.com/ya7o2qrb
18. tinyurl.com/yapfa3rh
19. tinyurl.com/y7tmjw7n
20. tinyurl.com/y83hyo46

16. Avoid Menopause Misery

1. tinyurl.com/yd23drpo
2. tinyurl.com/yddt7yyb
3. Ibid.
4. Ibid.
5. "Natural Medicines in the Clinical Management of Menopausal Symptoms," Clinical Management Series, NMCD Website, subscription required, tinyurl.com/ycj6lcsv.
6. Ibid.
7. Ibid.
8. Ibid.
9. Ibid.
10. Adapted from: tinyurl.com/y75gvmdp
11. Ibid.
12. tinyurl.com/y9tbe8lj
13. Adapted from: Ibid
14. tinyurl.com/y75gvmdp

17. Sleep Sounder

1. tinyurl.com/y3qm8nmp
2. tinyurl.com/yauly49w
3. Adapted from: tinyurl.com/ycxc96ln
4. tinyurl.com/yxoq8wgn
5. tinyurl.com/yahocygb
6. tinyurl.com/y7ar279t
7. tinyurl.com/y8m7gz6k
8. tinyurl.com/y964fo89
9. tinyurl.com/y5g5mrf7
10. tinyurl.com/y7d2yy2t
11. tinyurl.com/y5x8quws
12. tinyurl.com/y5whumvo
13. tinyurl.com/y762cenr
14. tinyurl.com/yauly49w
15. tinyurl.com/y9tfhy3y
16. tinyurl.com/yafe3kol

17. tinyurl.com/yb79u5q3
18. tinyurl.com/y8seazgt
19. Adapted from: tinyurl.com/y4my3mqj
20. Ibid.
21. tinyurl.com/yxorzhsf
22. Adapted from: tinyurl.com/yaqxt6pb
23. Adapted from: Ibid.
24. tinyurl.com/y7kjnlrm
25. tinyurl.com/ycgjvy48
26. tinyurl.com/y7arcwup
27. tinyurl.com/y76e2ojv
28. tinyurl.com/y6vgxj5u
29. tinyurl.com/yx8orbah
30. tinyurl.com/yb6pk3yp
31. tinyurl.com/y7y42tqm
32. tinyurl.com/y7wfc2bc
33. tinyurl.com/ya9hyokg
34. Ibid.
35. Ibid.
36. tinyurl.com/ybeg6fjq
37. tinyurl.com/yb6wo5ve
38. Ibid.
39. "Natural Medicines in the Clinical Management of Insomnia," Clinical Management Series, NMCD Website, subscription required, tinyurl.com/ycj6lcsv.
40. Ibid.
41. Ibid.

18. Protect Your Skin

1. tinyurl.com/yde6pes7
2. Adapted from: tinyurl.com/zjzplpp
3. tinyurl.com/ybsglt7r
4. tinyurl.com/y7aozlet
5. tinyurl.com/yboc7klk
6. tinyurl.com/y7nsbl5w
7. tinyurl.com/hlg3nwt
8. Adapted from: Ibid.
9. tinyurl.com/n3hjrgm
10. tinyurl.com/ya5l4ty5
11. Ibid.
12. Ibid.
13. tinyurl.com/y9qvwzmy

SPIRITUAL HEALTH TIPS

19. 12 Steps for Spiritual Strength Training

1. John Ortberg, *The Life You've Always Wanted: Six Sessions on Spiritual Disciplines for Ordinary People* (Grand Rapids, MI: Zondervan, 2004), 20.
2. tinyurl.com/yd7mmzve
3. tinyurl.com/yd9hxkfy
4. Ibid.
5. tinyurl.com/y93h9pvd
6. tinyurl.com/y2c2vtz3, tinyurl.com/yxaedx9j
7. tinyurl.com/y5hwb4sw
8. tinyurl.com/y5vxasad
9. tinyurl.com/y8xqfzx8
10. Ibid.

20. Develop an Attitude of Gratitude

1. tinyurl.com/y634h4xv
2. tinyurl.com/y6le5ol6
3. tinyurl.com/yaJt5mJb
4. tinyurl.com/y5plzcrl, tinyurl.com/y6svkqrn

21. Read More—Especially the Bible

1. tinyurl.com/y6sotat3
2. Ibid.
3. Ibid.
4. tinyurl.com/yyot2jqs
5. tinyurl.com/opanqmc
6. tinyurl.com/yxkjhv82
7. tinyurl.com/yxdzt8p4
8. tinyurl.com/y9aarvjp
9. Ibid.
10. Ibid.
11. tinyurl.com/y7u7g3yr
12. tinyurl.com/yc5osmzu
13. Quoted from: Ibid.
14. Ibid.
15. Ibid.
16. tinyurl.com/yaah5kcy
17. Ibid.
18. tinyurl.com/ycy6tb3d
19. tinyurl.com/yaah5kcy
20. Scott Bolinder, personal communication, November 13, 2018.
21. K.W. Oliver, *God's Handbook: Learn to Use the Bible to Answer All of Life's Most Difficult Questions!* (Five O' Eight Publishing, 2015).
22. Charles F. Stanley, *Handbook for Christian Living: Biblical Answers to Life's Tough Questions* (Nashville, TN: Thomas Nelson, 2008).
23. tinyurl.com/y7scekzo
24. Robert Chapman, "What the Bible Contains," *The Sunday School Journal and Bible Student's Magazine* (Thomas B. Neely, Editor) xxxv, no 8 (1903): 535. Also found in "The Wonderous Book," *The Epworth Herald: A Magazine for Young People and Older People with Younger Hearts* (Joseph Berry, Editor) XIV, no. 30 (December 26, 1903): 770(6).

22. Meditate and Pray

1. tinyurl.com/y7fkbt54
2. tinyurl.com/ycxywzcx
3. tinyurl.com/y58knfvr
4. tinyurl.com/y42srxme, tinyurl.com/y2feemka
5. tinyurl.com/y4uxsbyn
6. Adapted from: tinyurl.com/y72duvox
7. tinyurl.com/y2phps8o
8. tinyurl.com/y2m74p5w
9. tinyurl.com/yaontunx
10. tinyurl.com/y9kvolzg
11. Ibid.
12. Phil heard Dr. Hendricks say this in a talk at the Harvey Hotel in Carrolton, Texas, in about 1987 and still remembers it clearly.
13. Attributed to Saint Teresa of Calcutta, tinyurl.com/yb7u3c75
14. Adapted from: tinyurl.com/y98bf6py
15. tinyurl.com/y62kdrtw
16. tinyurl.com/y2me3hsb

RESOURCES BY WALT LARIMORE, MD

Books on Health

10 Essentials of Highly Healthy People:
Becoming and Staying Highly Healthy

Alternative Medicine: The Christian Handbook
(with Dónal O'Mathuúna)

God's Design for the Highly Healthy Person (with Traci Mullins)

God's Design for the Highly Healthy Teen (with Mike Yorkey)

God's Design for the Highly Healthy Child
(with Stephen and Amanda Sorenson)

The Highly Healthy Child (with Traci Mullins)

Lintball Leo's Not-So-Stupid Questions About Your Body
(with John Riddle)

SuperSized Kids: How to Rescue Your Child from the
Obesity Epidemic (with Sherri Flynt and Steve Halliday)

The Ultimate Guy's Body Book

The Ultimate Girl's Body Book (with Amaryllis Sánchez Wohlever)

Why ADHD Doesn't Mean Disaster
(with Dennis Swanburg and Diane Passno)

Web Resources

www.DrWalt.com

www.DrWalt.com/blog

www.Devotional.DrWalt.com

To learn more about Harvest House books and
to read sample chapters, visit our website:

www.harvesthousepublishers.com

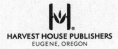

HARVEST HOUSE PUBLISHERS
EUGENE, OREGON